SUNSET ANGELS

A Companion Guide for New Hospice Nurses

Ellen G. Morgan, RN, BSN, CHPN

Cover and interior design by Kaycee Parker: www.kpcommunications.net

E-book ISBN: 979-8-9918804-1-1
Paperback ISBN: 979-8-9918804-0-4

I lovingly dedicate this book to my parents, Concordio and Fausta Simpliciano, who taught me the meaning of perseverance.

I also dedicate this book to all the hospice team members I have worked with at Capital Caring Team 1007, Goodwin House Hospice, and Asante Hospice. Without them, I would not have had these experiences to share with those of you who want to join this sacred work.

CONTENTS

INTRODUCTION

Congratulations on taking a huge step if you've just been hired as a hospice RN case manager!

If you have been seriously considering entering hospice, this book was also written for you.

I've been a hospice nurse for over ten years, and I can't think of another area of nursing I'd rather be in. I'm so glad you have entered into this nursing specialty. Yes, some days can be difficult, but every day is different and comes with its own challenges.

Hospice will stretch and grow you in ways you never thought possible.

This is just the beginning of your hospice career. You have now been given the chance to come alongside patients and family members at a very delicate and difficult time in their lives. You can potentially make a huge and memorable impact. If you are up to that challenge, then you have entered into the right field. I took that challenge many years ago, and it has changed me for the better.

I wish the same for you and want to cheer you on!

Because hospice is the care of the dying, it is not an area that nurses are drawn to in droves. It can be scary and intimidating. It is not different from entering into any other specialty in medicine—like cardiology, radiology, oncology, etc. You are stepping into an area of nursing that is critically needed in our communities. With the increasing numbers of an aging population, the need for hospice nurses is also rising. In this year of 2024 alone, every day, more than 11,000 Americans will reach the age of sixty-five.

This book has a specific purpose. It is to inform and equip nurses like you, who are new to hospice, and to prepare you for what's ahead. It's meant to take away some of the guesswork of what's coming and alleviate your fears about it.

When I was orienting new nurses, it was very discouraging to see them quit after only a few months. One in particular comes to my mind. Her name was Jeanette, and I thought she would have been an excellent hospice nurse. I helped orient her, but she left shortly after completing orientation. I was so heartbroken that she left our company. *We shouldn't be losing good nurses like this*, I said to myself.

This book was borne out of the desire to help nurses like Jeanette and to help you survive and thrive in the world of hospice. I believe in hospice work and want you to stay in it for as long as you can or desire. I believe we can make a huge difference and contribute to society through our work. I hope this book will show you what to expect in the coming weeks and months of your new job.

I have taken the time to really think back about the things that were helpful to me when I first started hospice. I've also included things I wish I had known back then to be better prepared for this work. You can use what I learned to your advantage now. I was recently talking with a new nurse on our team. She was a seasoned nurse in her forties and had come to hospice after working in other areas of nursing. She was glad to be on our team but said, "You never really know what to expect in hospice." I've heard that many times before from new nurses.

In the following chapters, I will go through a lot of information that might feel overwhelming at first. I would advise you not to read this book in one sitting, but instead to take your time. Read it as you go along during your hospice orientation. It may reinforce what you learn or bring up questions you want to ask.

I envisioned and wrote this book in a workbook fashion to be interactive and thought-provoking for you. At the end of each chapter, I've asked questions and provided space to write out your thoughts on what you've just read. This was designed to help you think and process the information given to you. I encourage you to take the time to answer those questions so you can get the most out of this book. If you have additional questions, be sure to ask the hospice team members you will be orienting with.

I encourage you to use this book as a reference or handbook. I can't tell you everything there is to know about hospice. That would be impossible, and I really don't want to overwhelm you in the beginning with all the details of this work.

I also would like to add that I am aware that there are new hospice nurses around the world and your experiences will be different in your country from my experiences here in the U.S. But my hope is that you can also take away and use the information presented in this book and tailor it to your needs.

The pages of this book contain my story—my journey, joys, and frustrations. Your journey will be different, but I want to help you get a good start by giving you a road map and direction to prepare you for what lies ahead. I've been where you are now and beyond. It was difficult to absorb it all in the beginning, but eventually, I took it all in, and you will, too. After a few weeks or even months of hospice work, the information you read in this book may start to make better sense, and you will fall into your own rhythm.

In the beginning, be patient with yourself and give yourself grace.

Being a hospice nurse is a beautiful experience. Yes, it has its difficulties, but overall, the satisfaction you will get from this work is indescribable. You will see for yourself in the weeks to come.

It took me a while to find a title for this book. I asked myself how I could capture the essence of what a hospice nurse does. I thought a sunset conveyed a sense of serenity and peacefulness. It's just what you would want a patient to experience at the end of their life. I cannot tell you how many times my patients or family members have called me and the nurses on our hospice team angels. So hence, the title *Sunset Angels* (caring for your patient at the end of their life). That's what you are.

I'm rooting for you as you embark on this new journey. I believe in you, and yes, you <u>can</u> do this!

CHAPTER 1

THE BIG QUESTION

Take a moment to ask yourself, "Why hospice, and why now?" That's the big question a former supervisor, Patty, asks during interviews with potential nurses. This may have been one of your interview questions. So, I want you to think back on your response, "What was your why?"

You might have had a close family member or friend in hospice services. You probably thought to yourself when watching the hospice nurse, *I wish I could do that.* Maybe you were impressed by how the hospice nurses took such good care of your loved one. A nurse colleague told me she became interested in hospice after her dad was in hospice care. You might have wanted to get into hospice work for a while because it intrigued you, and a position opened up, so you applied for it.

Whatever your reason for going into hospice, it was a courageous step for you to take. It is an area in nursing that is so vitally needed. When people say it takes a special kind of person to be a hospice nurse, it's true. Guiding patients and their families through probably the darkest time in their lives takes a very brave person. Not everyone can do this kind of work.

Right now, you might be asking yourself, what does it take to be a good hospice nurse? The qualities of kindness, patience, gentleness, and compassion come quickly to mind. But really and truly, I've seen every personality type. Some are soft-spoken introverts, and others are outgoing and sociable. Both can succeed in hospice. I believe if you have the drive, passion, and determination to learn to help others through this most difficult time in their lives, then you have the potential to be an excellent hospice nurse.

I've thought back to my own journey into hospice, which took a meandering path. I had a taste of it early on in my nursing career. In my third year of nursing, after I gave birth to our first baby girl, I wanted to stay home with her longer than the six weeks of maternity leave I had available. So, I applied for an on-call or (PRN) position at a hospice company. The position was affiliated with the hospital I worked for, so it was a fairly easy transition. I was tasked with covering for the RN case managers when they went on vacation. I did it for about nine months and thought it was a pretty interesting job. It was a short stint in hospice, but I knew in the back of my mind that I wanted to do it again sometime later in my career. Afterward, I returned to hospital work as a float nurse, worked in the renal/dialysis unit, and did some critical care work.

A few years later, I left the hospital and entered into other areas of nursing, like home care, telephonic disease management, and school nursing, and I also worked in a long-term care facility.

Then, in my nineteenth year of nursing, I had the opportunity to return to hospice. My family moved from Indiana to Virginia, and I was looking for a job. We went to church one Saturday and were invited to the pastor's house for lunch. As it turned out, his wife was a clinical supervisor for a hospice company in northern Virginia. She encouraged me to apply for an RN case manager position, which I did. She said she would look out for my application to "help" it go through the process faster. And the rest, as they say, is history.

As you can see, I've worked in many areas of nursing, which is an advantage of being a nurse. The areas you can work in are very diverse. I've applied all the knowledge I have learned over the years to my hospice work.

But enough about me, let's go back to you.

So here you are, about to start your new hospice job. What now? You must have a lot of questions going through your mind on what to expect in this area of nursing. You may be wondering; *can I really do this?* Or, *what am I getting myself into? Am I going to like it?* I want you to know that I also had those thoughts, doubts, and fears. I can now confidently say, yes, it is possible; you *can* do it and succeed.

You are capable of doing so much good in hospice.

I also want you to know that you are a very valuable person on your hospice team. Your administrators chose you for a reason. They saw something(s) in you that made you a good fit for hospice work.

At the start of this chapter, I mentioned Patty, a former supervisor, and her "why" question. I've asked her what compels her to want to hire a nurse during her interview process. She said she looks for someone who has been drawn to hospice in some way. They must be articulate "as families will be hanging on their every word." She looks for someone who is organized in their work. She also seeks individuals who have a level of confidence in talking with patients and families. Finally, she looks for someone who is eager to learn because "people really have no clue of all that is required for a nurse to know in hospice." This is so true.

Like I said before, not everyone can do this work. Because you were chosen, know that you have the skills and ability to do this hospice work, even if you don't believe it right now. When I first started, I sure didn't. But go ahead, take another courageous step forward. I'm rooting for you all the way!

THOUGHTS AND NOTES:

What thoughts and questions are going through your mind about hospice now? What do you hope to learn in this work as a hospice nurse? Write your questions here and ask your hospice team members about them during orientation. Think of one or two goals you would like to accomplish in the next week as you start your orientation, and write it down, too. Make it simple, nothing too hard.

GOALS:

"What you get by achieving your goals is not as important as what you become by achieving your goals." - Zig Ziglar

Shortly after I started hospice, our team had a family meeting with a large family whose grandmother was very precious to them. One said she was "The center of all of us." I felt so much love in the room as we discussed how to best care for her. It was an honor to experience this early on in my hospice career, and I remember it fondly, even now. This case reminded me that I should consider every patient as precious because that person is a treasure to someone.

SUNSET MEMORY

CHAPTER 2

BUILD YOUR KNOWLEDGE BASE

In your first year of hospice nursing, strive to learn as much as you can about this work. This is not like any other nursing position you have had before. During orientation, watch and observe how things are done, and ask questions to every team member you orient with. It could be the hospice chaplain, social worker, your nurse case manager colleagues, and even your hospice medical director (HMD) or nurse practitioner. This is a job where you will be out in the field, whether at a patient's home or visiting a patient in a facility.

One thing that was helpful to me in the beginning was getting a small notebook, which I kept in my work folder (I still have one). I briefly wrote down important things or observations I learned during my workdays. These were short notes to myself, not journaling, for which I had a separate book. In it, I would also write down anything that would help me do my work well. These included tips from watching other nurses and what to do and what not to do. It gave me a place to write down my thoughts right away so I wouldn't forget the information, and I could refer to it later on when I needed it. The first hospice doctor I worked with, Dr. Shariff, would give me some very useful medical tips when visiting patients with him. These were things he learned in medical school and his own hospice experience, which he passed on to me and the other nurses on our team.

The following are the topics you'll be covering during orientation:

1. Pain management - As a hospice nurse, you are expected to provide comfort to your patients, and a large part of that is knowing what medications would be effective in relieving different types of pain:

nociceptive, neuropathic, or visceral pain. When calling your HMD, learn how to manage pain effectively and ask questions if you are not sure. Familiarize yourself with all the pain meds you will use to manage patients' pain well. This is not something you will learn in just a few weeks, but during orientation, learn as much as you can about pain management with meds as well as non-pharmacological ways to provide comfort. This will be an ongoing learning topic for you during your hospice nursing career.

2. Time management - This is an essential skill that you will need to master to be efficient in your workday. During orientation, when making visits with your nurse colleagues, you will be learning how to plan your visits at the beginning of the day and how to be aware of your time throughout the day so you can accomplish what you need to. There are also recertification reports and interdisciplinary team (IDT) notes to complete, which you will learn how to do. There may be face-to-face (F2F) visits, and you may need to accompany your hospice medical director (HMD) or nurse practitioner (NP) if this is your company's requirement. So, you will need to organize all these items for your caseload. I go into more detail about this in Chapter 8.

3. Learning your Electronic Medical Record (EMR) system - This is your company's documentation system and is something you are required to know for your daily charting. Make it a goal to be efficient with charting while you are in orientation. You will avoid a lot of frustration when you're out on your own if you focus on this. Try your best to master your EMR system as much as you can during the coming weeks. You won't know fully until you are doing visits on your own, but at least you will have a good foundation from which to start.

4. Collaborating and communicating with your hospice team members - Remember that even if you are out in the field, you have a hospice team you can communicate with. The more you keep in touch with your team members, the more effective you will be in caring for your patients. I have elaborated on this topic in Chapter 7.

5. Using effective communication methods with patients, families, and facility staff to promote trust - There are so many ways to build trusting relationships with people, which you probably already know. The one thing I've learned about communication in hospice is that more is better. If you overcommunicate with your patients, it's much better than not communicating enough with them. Developing trust in your work is key to your success.

Remember, every new hospice nurse has been where you are. If you forget how to do something, ask your team members. I'm sure your clinical supervisor and nurse colleagues will be happy to assist you. During orientation, keep asking lots of questions because if you don't ask them now, you'll be asking them later on. Keep writing important things in your little notebook because many things will fly over your head if you don't write them down. At the end of the day, take a quick five to ten minutes to review your notes. Hopefully, this will help you retain what you've learned. And if you forget, keep asking those questions.

One very important tip I wish I had known is to take the time to focus on this work by simplifying my life. As you may have already imagined, it is going to take a lot out of you, emotionally and physically. Avoid taking on anything new during these next few months. Streamline your responsibilities at home so you can focus on learning this skill of hospice.

If you have a family, discuss how to best delegate housework to make your home routine more manageable. Tell them that this job is going to require teamwork from them. Warn them that you need to make some changes so that you can succeed in this work. This is something that I really wished someone had told me to do when I first started hospice. Instead, I tried to do it all and be a super mom and a super nurse. But that was impossible and really did not work for me and my family. I wish I had taken the time to make my family aware of what I needed and to ask what they needed from me. It would have prevented a lot of stress and strain. Have these discussions and regularly check in with your family, whether weekly or monthly. Do what works for you. Be sure to plan family activities together, just to be with them and have fun so that your focus is not all about work.

If you are single or married with no children, I believe this tip can apply to you too. Take the time to make your life simpler because this work will take up a lot of space in your life at first. Later, when you become skilled at your work, you'll have more time to do other things.

Another tip for building your knowledge of hospice is having a mentor. The first hospice company I worked for had mentors for new nurses during orientation. I was assigned to a mentor named Sheila Lax, a seasoned hospice nurse. I can still hear her talking in her proper British accent. In my first few weeks and months, she took me under her wing and showed me how to do hospice.

The following is a blog I wrote about a memorable experience I had with Sheila:

> *"I remember well the days when I would meet at her home during the first weeks of hospice orientation. As we started our morning talk, she would offer me a cup of tea. As I sipped the warm tea she made for me, I learned my first lesson. I was usually one who was too impatient to sit down and drink a full cup of tea. I was too eager to get about doing things. Back then, I would go from one task to another with no breaks in between. Sheila taught me to stop—take a breath and rest a bit. She was so gracious to invite me to her home—neat and tastefully decorated. I felt refreshed when I stepped into her living room. Her home was peaceful and calm, and it helped me quiet my spirits."*

Sheila had a wealth of knowledge about hospice that she did not hold back from sharing. I sensed that she had a healthy outlook on her work, and I wanted that. She was always willing to answer my many questions and give me good advice. And at the end of each talk, she would say, "Now, go out there and make a difference!" She continued to be supportive as the years went by. Having a mentor to guide me through those early years and having her as a sounding board was so valuable to me.

Not all hospice company orientations are the same. So, ask your clinical supervisor if they have mentors for new nurses. If they do, you will have that person as a resource and support as you transition into hospice work. If not, you will have your fellow RN case manager colleagues who will help orient and guide you. If you want some consistency, choose the one(s) you like best or feel the most comfortable with. Ask them whether they would agree to be a mentor or a "go-to" person when you have questions or are in a bind. Most nurses will try to be accommodating, so don't be afraid to ask. Your clinical supervisor, who was likely an RN case manager before, can also be a great resource and is very knowledgeable. Everyone has been where you are right now—at the very beginning. It's ok to feel afraid and a little anxious. I know I was.

For me, the first year of hospice was exciting, scary, and intimidating all at the same time. I didn't know exactly what I was getting into. But I had a great team to work with, and that made a huge difference. Your first year can be a great learning experience for you too. I am confident that you will learn this work if you consistently put effort into it.

The one resource your clinical supervisor will probably give you is the booklet Hospice *Quickflips© for NGS: A Guide for Clinicians by Corridor*[1]. It is a teaching tool for RN case managers about documentation and hospice eligibility. It is easy to read and contains useful information that you will refer to over and over again.

[1] Corridor Hospice Quickflips© - NGS https://a.co/d/5KtEYIz

THOUGHTS AND NOTES:

How will you make time and space in your life to learn this new skill of hospice nursing? Write down your plan and give it a try. If it needs adjusting later, tweak it until you free up more time for this work.

"Life is not easy for any of us. But what of that? We must have perseverance and, above all, confidence in ourselves. We must believe that we are gifted for something and that this thing must be attained." - Marie Curie

When we moved to Oregon and were in orientation with a new hospice company, I did visits with our chaplain, Richard, for a day. He was a gregarious Englishman who was a lot of fun to do visits with. I watched and learned as he went from patient to patient, taking the necessary time to listen to each one. He stressed the importance of being present with them and providing what he could to meet their emotional needs.

SUNSET MEMORY

CHAPTER 3

THE PROS OF HOSPICE

When you look at the pros and cons of this work, you might think there are many more cons than pros. If you dwell on the negative aspects of hospice, you will find many. On the other hand, if you choose to focus on the positives of your work, you will find them and be more likely to stay in it. One of the reasons why I asked you in the first chapter to think about why you decided to get into hospice is to keep you focused on the good things —the positive things that will carry you through the difficult times.

If I were to ask you what the pros of hospice are, what would they be for you? The following things have been pros for me. Some I noticed right when I started and others later as I got more into the work. See if you can relate and maybe add to my list.

- *You are the master of your days as a case manager.* If you like working independently and feel confident doing so, this will be a real plus for you. You can plan your own work schedule and make adjustments as things come up. As you plan your weekly patient visits, you can tailor them to your life. You are, to a large extent, the boss of your work. You have the freedom to change and adjust your day to work for you. But I need to warn you that even with all your careful planning, things may not go exactly how you expected them to, so stay flexible throughout your day.

This was and still is the biggest perk and what I love about hospice. The autonomy of this job is what keeps me in it.

- *You are not required to work evening or night shifts.* Case management is a day shift job. In the hospital, the night shift was my least favorite one to work, and the evening shift kept me away from my family, which I didn't like. Working weekends in hospice may or may not be mandatory. Some companies require you to work on-call shifts, but at least you get to choose what days you want to work. The weekend work requirement varies with each hospice company.

For example, in the first hospice company I worked for, it was mandatory for us to choose our on-call for weekends and some weekday evenings. At the second company, it was not mandatory to do weekend on-call. It was encouraged but not mandatory. My supervisor would email us the needs for the weekends, and we would choose whether we wanted to work or not. The hospice company I work for now requires occasional "backup" weekends throughout the year, but these days are ones you can choose.

- *You can choose your holidays to work.* Toward the end of the year, your supervisor will email you to choose the holidays you want to work in the upcoming year. Most companies ask that you choose a major and a minor holiday to work. Since you are new, your supervisor may or may not ask you to pick up holidays, depending on the time of the year you are hired. This is something you might want to ask your supervisor about. I always made sure that when I saw this holiday schedule email from my supervisor, I would send in my choices quickly because it's usually first come, first served. And just like the hospital, you are compensated with an increase in your pay when you work on holidays, which is a nice incentive.

- *You can attend your children's school events if you have a family.* This was a huge plus for me. The RNCM positions I had were salary positions, not paid hourly. So, if I needed to take some time off for my family or doctor appointments, I would just need to make prior arrangements with my supervisor, preferably a week ahead of time or more. If I had school events to attend during the day or early evening, I would let my supervisor know ahead of time. In addition, my responsibility was to ask another nurse to cover for me for the hour or two I would be gone.

- *You are home for dinner with your family in the evenings.* A hospice nurse case manager's job usually starts at 8 a.m. and ends at 5 p.m. It was important for me to be home, make dinner, and spend time with my family, so the day shift hours really appealed to me.

- *Some companies pay year-end bonuses.* At the two hospice companies I worked for in Virginia, there was a year-end incentive bonus connected to individual performance and the team's overall performance. These were usually given in December, which really came in handy for the holidays. After all the hard work I'd done throughout the year, this was a bonus to look forward to. Find out if your company offers this kind of incentive or something similar.

- *Hospice work can grow you in your personal life if you allow it to.* It has certainly changed my whole outlook on things. I know what's really important to me in my life. I've learned to nurture and take good care of myself. It's still a work in progress, but I'm making more time to do so. I know when to ask for help. I know when to stop over-obsessing with details and have fun. I'm trying not to take myself too seriously and enjoy life more fully. All of this takes work, and if it wasn't for hospice, I don't think I would have grown, matured, and become the person I am today.

- *You will meet and care for some really fascinating people during your hospice career.* I've known scientists, military veterans, lawyers, doctors, artists, engineers, etc. I've even cared for a patient who has been to all seven continents in the world. And as you get to know your patients, you will learn valuable life lessons from each one. It's amazing to see how each patient has used their skills and talents to significantly impact their community. I remember a woman who had a doctorate in chemistry. During one of my visits, she pointed to a book she wrote on the shelf. She said, "People tend to forget our contributions to society." I am guilty of this, and it has increased my appreciation and respect for the elderly. Many of them have lived very successful and productive lives.

This is another of the top reasons why I remain in hospice. Both patients and family members have taught me lessons that are like jewels to me. They have enriched my life in so many ways.

- *This is obvious, but the knowledge you learn as a hospice nurse will help you personally when a family member or friend goes into hospice.* It will not be a mystery. You will know what to expect and do. You will be able to help guide your family and friends on their final journey toward the end of their lives.

This list will become important to you when the days get tough and when the work becomes challenging. With this list, you can see the reasons why you got into hospice to remind yourself of the positive things about it.

THOUGHTS AND NOTES:

Are there things you have already seen about hospice that are pros for you? Write your own list here. Ask the other hospice nurses what they like about their job; add them to your list if you like.

"Whatever good things we build end up building us." - Jim Rohn

Before we left Virginia, I was scheduled to see one of my Middle Eastern patients. His daughter asked me not to forget to see her father one last time, so I made sure to see him. At the end of my visit, she said they had something to give me. Her family thanked me for caring for their father and handed me a package. She said that she had special ordered it from the Middle East, where they were from, so I knew it was special. When I got home, I opened it, and it was a beautifully embroidered dark teal and olive bedspread with coral-colored lotus flowers tastefully stitched throughout. It took my breath away and brought tears to my eyes. I will always treasure this gift.

SUNSET MEMORY

CHAPTER 4

GIVE YOURSELF TIME

I encourage you to allow ample time to master hospice so that you will know if it is truly an area of nursing that fits you.

In hospice, you will learn a new culture, language, and way of thinking as a nurse. You will move from a "curative" to a "comfort" mindset. When I started working at my first hospice job, a social worker friend and former colleague, Joyce, told me to try it for three years to give it a real chance. I would tend to agree. But if you are not sure you want to commit three years of your life to hospice, I would ask that you consider staying in it for a year. Personally, the first year was really the toughest one since everything was new to me.

In the first six months, I felt like I was in unfamiliar territory, and not really knowing what to expect, it took some time to formulate my rhythm and routine. I tried my hardest to keep my head above water in the following six months. In these months, you, too, will experience many difficult things. I remember the challenges and tough situations with patients and families when I first started. Those are the times when you really need to lean on your team. Their experience will help carry you through those times. If you view these challenges as learning points instead of pass-or-fail events, then every experience will build upon the other, and you will become a stronger nurse.

Another term for this is called emotional courage. Merriam-Webster defines courage as a "mental or moral strength to venture, persevere, and withstand danger, fear, or difficulty." In his book Leading with Emotional Courage, author Peter Bregman describes emotional courage as "The courage to feel. It's what stands between us and the difficult things we must do . . ." Emotional courage grows stronger when you practice it—by taking a risk, making a decision, or otherwise following through when you may not be comfortable doing so." ChatGPT gave this definition of emotional courage: It "refers to the ability to confront and manage difficult emotions or situations with resilience, honesty, and vulnerability. It involves facing fears, expressing oneself authentically, and navigating emotional challenges with strength and integrity."

Personally, I think *emotional courage* is an important characteristic that all hospice nurses need because of the work they do.

If you take the time to learn, grow, and adapt to this hospice work, you will be equipped to help patients and families work through their difficult issues. Flexibility and the willingness to learn are two other traits that will help you be successful in your work.

If you can survive the first year, navigating your ship through the rough waters of this job, you will have accomplished a great deal. In the second year, you will begin to feel more confident and know what to do when you go through storms and challenges. Then, by the third year, you'll truly feel like the captain of your ship. By the time the third year rolled around, I felt more self-assured and wasn't as anxious about new or difficult situations as I used to be. By then, I had a lot of experience under my belt. That was my journey. Of course, yours will be different.

This one-year commitment is just my recommendation, my own opinion. I share this because I've seen too many new hospice nurses quit shortly after orientation. Whether you choose to stay in hospice is totally your choice, but I encourage you to stick it out for at least a year and then decide whether to stay or not. If you have a supportive team, you will be more likely to have a positive experience the longer you are in it.

THOUGHTS AND NOTES:

I really want you to be successful in your hospice work, and believe me, it will take time. What time commitment will you choose to fully learn this work? Six months? A year or beyond?

Remember those goals you wrote down in Chapter 1? Have you made any progress? Write how you have reached your goals. Or are they still a work in progress? Do you have any new goals?

"Success is the sum of small efforts, repeated day in and day out." - Robert Collier

I recently talked to Audrey, one of our team RNCMs. She said our HMD had complimented her, and she said, "I've been in hospice for about two and a half years, and at times I still feel new and have impostor syndrome." She said sometimes she doesn't feel like a real hospice nurse. It was surprising to hear Audrey say this because I think she is a very caring and conscientious nurse to her patients. And they love her. It doesn't matter whether a nurse is starting in hospice or has been in it for a while; there may still be doubts and wonder about whether they are "good enough." I have felt inadequate from time to time. But that's okay. It's all part of the learning process.

SUNSET MEMORY

CHAPTER 5

YOUR HOSPICE COMPANY

The success of your hospice career largely depends on the company you work for. Not all hospice companies operate the same way. How they care for you will affect your longevity in hospice. I hope you looked at the reviews of the company that hired you. Did the nurses feel respected for their time, health, and well-being? Or did they make unreasonable work demands on them? The caseload (the number of patients you're assigned) that you are given will also determine whether you stay in hospice for the long term or not. The ideal caseload is eleven to fourteen patients. These numbers can vary from urban areas to rural areas. Keep in mind that your hospice census will rise and fall like waves. Don't be surprised if your caseload climbs to sixteen or seventeen during those busy times. Then, you might have a low caseload after several of your patients die or are discharged. In the beginning, your supervisor may start you off with a caseload of six to eight patients, depending on your company policy.

This may also vary according to the region of the country you are working in. But generally, this is a manageable caseload for a new hospice nurse. Over time, your caseload will increase as you tell your clinical supervisor that you are comfortable taking on more patients. You need to let your clinical supervisor know your comfort level, or they will assume you're ok with it. Speak up if you are getting overwhelmed. If you don't tell them, they won't know. And avoid comparing yourself to the other new nurses. Take your time and go slow. Take on what you can handle. Keep communicating with your clinical supervisor about what is going well and what is not for you. Once you feel competent, and that day will come, you will be a stronger nurse and well-equipped to take on more patients.

While you are on orientation, ask the other RN case managers about their caseloads. What are their numbers? What's the highest caseload they've ever had? This will give you an idea of what your company's expectations of you are. Also, ask your nurse colleagues about the company's culture. You can learn a lot from different companies. If you find out the RNCM's caseloads are high, I encourage you to still move forward with the job. Learn as much as you can, but know that high caseloads are not sustainable, and, at some point, you may say you are not willing to put yourself through that much stress. That would be the time to start looking for another hospice position elsewhere.

The first hospice company I worked for required their nurses to have caseloads of nineteen and upward into the twenties. At one time, I had twenty-nine patients. During my first year, I tried everything I could to adjust to this caseload and make it manageable, but it was a constant struggle. If they had an admission for me to do in the middle of the day, I couldn't say no; I just had to do it. That was the mentality and the culture of the company. I didn't have a work-life balance, and my family relationships suffered. I was tired and exhausted all the time. I hung on for five years, but it was not manageable in the long term, and I finally had to get out. The only reason why I stayed so long was because of my very caring hospice team. We really had a strong bond and did life together. It was hard to leave them, but it came down to choosing between my work and my health. I was burned out and needed a mental break. Looking back on this initial hospice position, I learned a lot about time management, teamwork, Alzheimer's and dementia, and how to care for wounds in hospice patients. It was a tough job, but it certainly gave me a good foundation in hospice.

A former RN case manager left our company to work for a smaller hospice company. I asked her if she was happy there, and she said she was, so I decided to give that company a try. This hospice company tried to keep their nurses' caseloads to about ten to fifteen patients. I was so glad I made the change. I was much happier, and my family was happier, too. I stayed four years with that company. The 2020 pandemic happened during that time, so I felt our team wasn't as close as my first team. But they were good years, and I felt I had more balance in my life. After leaving that team, I realized that hospice nursing is the same wherever you are. Whether you have a smaller or higher caseload, you still need to consciously care for yourself. You can easily burn out in this work if you are not deliberately nurturing yourself. I would say your success in hospice is 60 percent related to your hospice company and 40 percent to your self-care. I will go further into that in the next chapter.

THOUGHTS AND NOTES:

What have the other RNCMs said about their caseloads? On average, how many do they have? How do they manage their caseloads? What do they do when they feel overwhelmed? Think about this expectation and how it will affect you.

I remember the farewell party that my first company's team members held for me. Joyce, one of our social workers, hosted this event in her warm and inviting home. I felt so loved and appreciated. I felt sad about leaving them, but I knew the decision I had made was a wise one for me. We had a fabulous time celebrating our past experiences together.

SUNSET MEMORY

CHAPTER 6

CARING FOR YOU EQUALS SUCCESS

Putting yourself first seems counterintuitive to many nurses, including myself. We always try to put others first and care for their needs before our own. However, caring for yourself well is one of the key elements of success in your job as a hospice nurse.

For the longevity of your time in hospice, it is crucial that you write out your self-care plan. If you think that sounds odd, I admit it seemed odd to me, too. Why should you do that? Let me tell you, if I don't write something down, it won't happen. I challenge you to be deliberate in knowing what you can handle as you care for yourself. No one else will do it for you. As nurses, we are natural givers; if we are not careful, we may give too much of ourselves, eventually leading to burnout. So, as you start your work in hospice, I suggest you write out how you will care for yourself while doing this work. Just as you have care plans for your patients, try to write a care plan to nurture yourself. Be realistic and create a plan that is doable for you. If this feels foreign, you're not alone. It is still a work in progress for me.

I do some things for self-care. Here is my list of things that refresh and revive me.

1. Going to Starbucks to enjoy a favorite or new drink. Sometimes, it's good for me to be in a different setting and just savor a warm drink.
2. Taking a walk. Exercise energizes me, and I always feel better after I have taken a walk.
3. Talking to a close friend. Talking things over helps me to de-stress.
4. Taking a power nap. I try to fit ten to twenty-minute naps into my day to energize me.

5. I enjoy reading a good book, even if only for five to ten minutes. I have also recently tried audiobooks and am learning a lot during my drives between patients.
6. Trying a new dinner recipe. I love being in the kitchen and creating something delicious.
7. Watching a good movie and eating popcorn with my husband.
8. Getting a manicure or pedicure. This makes me feel polished and put together.
9. Crocheting. This mindless craft helps me not to think of work, and I get to create something beautiful at the same time.
10. Taking pictures of nature and making picture cards. It makes me happy to give them to others.
11. I close my eyes and take deep tummy breaths. When I exhale, I feel calmer and less anxious.
12. Making a healthy smoothie. This always makes me feel good inside.
13. Going to a new shop I have seen and wanted to go to. Sometimes, I like window shopping and looking for creative art or ideas.

I used to think this was enough for me. But I recently read a book called *The Self-Care Prescription: Powerful Solutions to Manage Stress, Reduce Anxiety, and Increase Well-being* by Dr. Robyn L. Gobin. She challenged my thoughts about what self-care really is. This is her definition of self-care:

> *"Simply put, self-care means taking care of yourself. But that means more than just treating yourself to occasional luxuries; it means taking responsibility for your well-being in all the important areas of your life. It involves spending dedicated time getting to know who you are and what you need to be happy, healthy, and fully present in your life."*

Dr. Gobin also stated that caring for your needs involves more than just doing fun activities. It also involves taking the time to self-reflect and figure out what works for you and what doesn't.

So, I came up with my own self-care list for being happy and healthy:

- I take multivitamins, including vitamin D (since my levels tend to be low), and oil of oregano capsules, which help boost my immune system and prevent colds.
- I try to eat healthy and stay away from processed foods as much as possible. Some days are better than others.
- Trying to get six or more hours of sleep per night.

- Trying to develop home systems so that I am efficient in my housework.
- Make time for myself. One hour per week to do something enjoyable.
- Do crafts so I can be creative.
- Exercise and watch my weight.
- Still working on realistic expectations.
- Wanting to make my life simpler.
- Trying to get rid of clutter.
- Trying to give myself grace instead of pushing so hard.
- I need to have time to sit and do nothing.
- Gardening has been my creative outlet. I enjoy watching my plants, flowers, and vegetables grow.
- I try to make time to process my work. I need to be more consistent with that. After charting, I journal for five to ten minutes to get work out of my head.
- I practice being concise with my charting so I can have more time with my family.

After I wrote this list, I realized I needed to be more self-aware. My life has been such a blur between raising a family and working, that I haven't made enough time for self-growth. I think this stems from always putting others first and me last. I've had to remind myself that making time for me is okay. And I felt better afterward, too. It may sound selfish, but what do you have to offer your patients if you are running on empty?

I can go on and on about self-care, self-love, nurturing, and nourishing yourself. I want you to be knowledgeable about self-care and do what works for you. Keep working at it because it will make you feel happier and more fulfilled.

Self-Care During Work

Let's shift gears a little and talk about caring for yourself during your workday. Hospice work requires a lot of energy, so caring for your physical body is essential. It may be easy to skip meals, but if you don't nourish your body, you won't be able to endure your work, and you will run out of steam faster than you would like. Pay attention to the meals you are eating. While it's nice to eat out when you are out in the field, time may not permit you to do that. And if you work in rural areas, you may not find fast-food places in the country. So, I suggest bringing your lunch. I usually bring leftovers from dinner or make a quick sandwich the night before to pack in my lunch bag in the morning.

There are lots of healthy foods you can bring for lunch. Some nurses even invest in a portable food warmer that you can hook up in your car to warm up stuff like leftover dinner, pizza, or just about anything that requires heating. If you have extra time to eat out, that's great. But generally, packing your lunch is an all-around better idea to save time and money. It is a huge plus if you can find a park or a quiet place to eat so you can unwind and enjoy some downtime while you eat. This may not always be possible, but it's a nice change of pace that will refresh you.

Staying hydrated is important, too. I never leave the house without my water thermos. Learn to find all the places you can stop for a restroom break. I make it a point to know where all the McDonald's are in my territory. Libraries are another place I stop for bathroom breaks. If I know I'm going to one of my facilities, I will drink more before I go there. I've seen some nurses ask if they could use their home patient's bathroom, but somehow, I can't get myself to do that.

I keep snacks in my nursing bag for days when I can't get to my lunch during long visits at a facility. For example, I remember a time when I had a long admission that took hours, and I was so hungry that I was on the verge of having a headache. Mike, one of our social workers, did the admission with me. He handed me a package of peanut butter cheese crackers that day while I was charting on our admission. I was so grateful for the snack. It kept me going until I could get to my lunch afterward. Those little things can carry you through hard days and help you keep going. From then on, I usually kept granola bars in my nursing bag just in case. Bring whatever you like to eat. It's nice to have an emergency snack.

Boundaries

As a case manager, creating boundaries helps other people, namely your patients and family members, know that you're not available 24/7. They will get attached to you, as you will to them, which is good. But it's also good to let them know that you are not available at all times of the day and night. Make those lines clear so that you are not running yourself ragged. You need and deserve time to rest and recuperate on evenings and weekends.

Creating boundaries also pertains to your workload. If you feel overwhelmed with your caseload of patients or are asked to do on-call when you are exhausted, let your supervisor know. If you say yes to everything to the detriment of your health, then you need to reevaluate your boundaries.

Phones

Part of having boundaries is training yourself to turn off your work phone after work hours and on the weekends. Some hospice companies will provide a separate work phone or may have you use your personal phone. If you use your personal phone for work, turn off the notifications or let your phone calls go to message if you see your patients trying to contact you. Remind your patients and families that an after-hours nurse will address concerns or issues outside your normal work hours. If they call in the middle of the night, resist the urge to answer the call. If they leave an urgent message, you can notify the after-hours nurse to let him/her know what your patient's needs are and ask them to call your patient.

I will admit that I have answered a family member's urgent call on a few occasions, but it isn't my usual routine. It's important to preserve your energy and get the rest you need after work and on weekends.

Turn Work Off

Blocking work out of your mind is a major skill to learn if you want to work in hospice for the long term. It is essential that you work on this skill until it becomes second nature to you. When you are done with your work, after you've finished charting at the end of the day or starting your weekend, make it a point to stop thinking and ruminating about the details of your work. That's when all the details will come to mind. All the things you think you should've done, could've done better, or worrying about patients and their families, etc. These things will flash through your mind. Let them go. These details will constantly invade your thoughts, taking away the mental energies that you should be using for rest and recovery.

For years, I thought about work almost constantly, trying to solve the problems of my patients and their families in my head. It literally drained me to the point of exhaustion. At the end of the week, I would be so tired that I would sleep for three hours on Saturday afternoons. People told me I looked tired all the time. One day, I decided I wasn't going to do that anymore. I made it a point to block work from my mind and mentally close the door on thoughts of work to get a break from it. In hospice, recovery is essential for your emotional well-being. I recommend that you make a point of learning how to do that right from the start.

Do not Suffer in Silence

During your orientation time, which may vary with different hospice companies, you will make visits with the other RNCMs on your team and other team members like social workers, chaplains, CNAs, etc. After orientation, you will be out in the field on your own. In the next few months, remember to reach out to your team members when you need help. Continue to ask them questions as they come up. I know how easy it is to feel alone once you're out there seeing patients by yourself. If you're not comfortable doing that yet, tell your supervisor. If you ask, your orientation time can be extended until you feel ready to work independently. If you are struggling with something, don't suffer in silence; don't try to wing it. Tell someone. Ask for help.

When you are ready to be out on your own, you will still have times of uncertainty and insecurity. Ask the questions you need to in order for you to feel competent. Speak up if you're not sure. Communicate with your clinical supervisor if you're having problems because no one will know what you're going through out in the field if you don't tell them. Don't suffer in silence; make your needs known.

Even as a seasoned hospice nurse, there have been times when I felt overwhelmed, even when my caseload was twelve to fifteen, which is supposed to be manageable. Sometimes, I had several wound care patients who literally took hours in my day to care for. So, the high acuity patients who need wound care, PleurX™ drains, patients who need ongoing symptom management, or those transitioning patients who are at the end-of-life (EOL) are the ones who will take up a lot of your time. Try your best to plan your week with a mixture of high and low-acuity patients so that you are not totally overwhelmed with all the challenging patients in one day. That's the beauty of being a case manager. You get to choose what your week will look like.

I remember having patients who needed extensive wound care, with visits taking over an hour. I would feel drained at the end of the day. I thought this was too much and talked to my supervisor. She empathized with me, and we discussed my caseload and pointed out how I could decrease my frequency of visits with other patients so that I could spend extra time with patients who really needed it. Afterward, I was able to breathe a sigh of relief. I was so glad to have had that time to brainstorm with her so we could make my workload more manageable. Call your supervisor, who can provide insight and guidance when your workload feels too heavy.

Another time you may feel the intensity of this work is when patients start to transition to end-of-life (EOL), which requires longer daily visits to manage symptoms. It can be hard to make the required visits for each patient. Depending on their needs, these EOL visits can easily take one to two hours. Again, don't suffer in silence. It will not benefit you at all. Tell your supervisor early in the day if you need help making your visits so arrangements can be made to help you. There might be another nurse whose caseload is low who can make visits for you.

Rest Periods

As you plan the hours of your days, intentionally incorporate breaks and lunch periods. It's so easy to plow through your day without any breaks in between because you want to get it all done. But you don't need to do it that way. Be consciously aware of what your physical needs are. Take those bathroom breaks. Take five- to ten-minute breathers to focus on your needs to have some sanity during the day. Take the time to eat your lunch. Or, if you're more of a grazer, bring nutritious snacks with you that you can eat throughout the day. Do what works for you to work and stay healthy.

Plan for Time off

In addition to having rest periods in your day, it's important to plan for vacations. This was a suggestion from a former bereavement counselor colleague, Dianne. I don't know when you can start taking vacations when you first start your job, maybe after six months or after getting through probation. Whatever your paid time off (PTO) or vacation time is structured with your company, I encourage you to look at the coming year and plan to take a day or two off every month. As a case manager, I didn't like to take too much time off, but looking back, I wish I'd done that differently.

Yes, we had our family vacations for about two weeks every summer, but I'm talking about the rest of the year. Try taking off a Friday or a Monday to have a three-day weekend. This can give you the additional physical and emotional rest you need. Maybe it's not every month; it could be every other month. Look at where the holidays fall and plan accordingly. You will have several paid holidays when you are off during the year. Be proactive and plan your vacations. The older I got, the more rest time I needed. It gave me more energy and desire to do my job well. So, take the time to plan ahead.

THOUGHTS AND NOTES:

Think of a self-care plan that will work for you personally and while you are doing hospice work. Write your plan here. Just do a quick outline and take more time later to elaborate.

Every morning, ask yourself, "What is one thing I will do today for self-care?" What will you do right now?

Today:

And how about weekly? What would be your self-care goal this week?

This week:

"Self-care is not selfish. You cannot serve from an empty vessel." - Eleanor Brown

When I first started hospice, I noticed one of our HMDs, Dr. S., would take time off every single month. He would attach his time off to a weekend to make it a three-day weekend. I admired that he intentionally took these mini vacations and wished I had done it myself.

Like my former hospice social worker, Mike, used to tell me, "Be good to yourself."

SUNSET MEMORY

CHAPTER 7

YOUR TEAM, YOUR SUPPORT

One of the major advantages of hospice nursing is that it's a team effort.

Your hospice team is made up of your executive director/manager, clinical supervisor, hospice medical directors, nurse practitioners, social workers, CNAs, bereavement counselors, and volunteer coordinators. Each one plays a vital role on your hospice team. Even though you are out in the field, you are only a phone call or text away from your teammates. As I've mentioned before, hospice nursing will take a lot out of you, physically and emotionally. If you feel like you're getting stuck with a patient, think of your other teammates and the support they can offer.

Again, I want to remind you that even though you're physically by yourself out there, you are never truly alone. Your team is there to help you.

Clinical Supervisor (CM)

Your clinical supervisor is there to oversee and guide you and the entire team, especially the RNCMs. Your supervisor is a valuable resource and can give you insight into other perspectives of problems you never thought of. I highly recommend that they be the first go-to person you reach out to when you have questions or difficult issues and don't know what to do. If you have a problem, your clinical supervisor will probably know the answer. If he or she doesn't, they will direct you to someone who does. They want you to be successful and will try their hardest to help you find the answers you need.

My first clinical supervisor, Grace, had an open-door policy, which was great for me as a newbie. In the beginning, I called her for just about anything I needed help with. She always took the time to brainstorm solutions to my problems. And it was just nice to talk through some difficult issues I couldn't solve on my own. Most clinical supervisors, including Grace, were case managers at one time. So, they know what you're going through.

Social Worker (SW)

Social workers are experts at providing emotional support for patients and their families. For families, it's often a very confusing and chaotic time when a loved one is dying. They discuss funeral arrangements and help patients and families choose one if they haven't already. They also help with legal issues or forms families need, like the Family and Medical Leave Act or letters requiring the hospice doctor's signature. These team members were also extremely helpful to me when I started hospice. They accompanied me when I did new admissions. Some hospice companies have nurses and social workers admit patients together, and others do not. There are pros and cons to both ways. You will learn about your company's procedures during orientation. If patients and families need help finding care at home, social workers will explore community resources appropriate to them.

Social workers help you with families with complex problems or issues with family dynamics. Some patients or family members may also be overly anxious or nervous about a particular issue. Social workers are usually able to spend more time working these issues out, so let them know and lean on them when this need arises.

Many Social workers are also trained counselors who can help you through your own issues regarding emotions about death and dying. I have relied heavily on my social workers while working as a hospice nurse. They have been my lifeline when I was caught in a difficult situation with work or personal issues. They have a wealth of knowledge they can share. I can remember times when my patients died, and I had a hard time processing the loss. I've sat down with a SW and had a mini-counseling session, which helped me tremendously.

Licensed Practical Nurses (LPNs)

Some hospices have LPNs on their teams, and some do not. I was fortunate to work closely with an LPN, Denise, while working for my first hospice company. That's when my caseload was nineteen and over. My highest number was twenty-eight. I would not have been able to keep up with my patient visits if it hadn't been for Denise's competent and efficient work. We would alternate seeing patients weekly, and that's how I was able to manage that high caseload. Plus, she was fun to work with. She had been with our company years before me and taught me a lot about hospice when I first started. If you have LPNs on your team, I encourage you to utilize their help to make your weekly visits.

Nurse Practitioner (NP)

Nurse practitioners are support people who can answer questions about your hospice work. I have worked with some great NPs. They do face-to-face (F2F) visits, which are done before recertifications (as described in Chapter 8). You may do joint F2F visits with them and learn from them. They actually welcome your help since you know your patients well. I have learned much by observing how they interact and care for my patients.

Another role they have is covering and taking your calls when the HMD is unavailable or on vacation. NPs have been valuable resources to me for answering questions or brainstorming patients' problems.

Hospice Medical Director (HMD)

Your team's HMD is also a great resource for you. However, their time is limited because they are busy overseeing all the nurses' calls on the team and more. So, your questions need to be focused before you call them. They do try their best to be available to answer your questions and teach you about different aspects of hospice.

I learned early on about hospice doctors, or at least the ones I've worked with, that they are very approachable. The ones I've known have been more than willing to teach nurses. After working with them, you will begin to feel like a true team player with your HMD. One of my former bereavement counselor colleagues said to me that hospice doctors are a different breed. In general, they are more open and will take the time to explain things so that you understand them.

When you have family meetings or a joint face-to-face (F2F) visit scheduled with the HMD, use that time to ask questions. I have asked many questions during F2F visits, which helped me add to my knowledge base as a hospice nurse.

The first HMD I worked with, Dr. Imran Shariff, was skilled at creating cohesiveness as a team. He also had a sense of humor, which, I think, is helpful in hospice so that you don't dwell on the sadness and dying part of hospice. He tried to keep our spirits up during our workdays. He was quick to answer any questions we had. He answered our calls and texts in a timely manner. We could depend on him and trust his judgment as he trusted ours.

Chaplain

Chaplains offer spiritual support to patients and their families. They are good listeners and can spend more time with a patient, listening and just being there for patients. There is much to be said about their presence with a dying patient. You can ask your chaplain to visit when your patient appears to be in spiritual and emotional distress. If a family requests last rites for their loved one, your chaplain can do that for them. Or if the family wants a specific clergy or a denominational minister to give last rites or prayers, they can make arrangements for them.

Chaplains can also offer you emotional support. I often used to call Arion, a former chaplain colleague, to help me process difficult patients or situations. We often talked about self-care. Not only did she listen to what I was going through, but she also encouraged me and lifted my spirits when I was feeling down about myself. She often asked me to do joint visits when seeing patients, and I enjoyed those visits with her.

Bereavement Counselor

These team members are trained grief counselors. They lead out with bereavement time, usually at the beginning of team IDT meetings when the team reviews and briefly discusses patients who have died since the last team meeting. They might even have a centering moment for the team, which may be an activity, poem, or short story. Bereavement counselors call family members, usually the patient's main caregiver, about four weeks after a patient has died to offer grief support. Their calls will continue for twelve months or until family members feel they no longer need this service.

Bereavement counselors not only help families process their grief, but they can also be a resource to help you figure out how to process complicated deaths. Especially the ones that don't make sense to you. Or the ones that linger in your mind that need grief work. Don't ignore those thoughts and feelings. In hospice, you will go through an array of feelings. You may experience sadness, grief, helplessness, hopelessness, disillusionment, guilt, etc. Throughout my hospice career, I have leaned on the wisdom of our bereavement counselors. They have helped me grow as a person and have made me an emotionally stronger person.

Hospice Aides

Hospice aides provide bathing and hygiene services to patients. Some hospice aides could also be Certified Nursing Assistants (CNAs). As an RN case manager, you will be required to supervise the hospice aides who care for your patients. Keep in touch with your them and instruct them to notify you of any changes they see in your patients. They are supposed to call you if they observe increased pain or agitation or notice any skin breakdown/wounds on your patients. I have often also called them to ask about a patient's meal/ food intake, mobility, and even their weight, if needed, for recertification reports. If a hospice aide is certified to do simple wound care, I have asked that hospice aide do the dressing changes on my busy days when I cannot make an extra visit. Hospice aides can also alert you when they see a patient declining and transitioning to end-of-life (EOL).

Volunteer Coordinator

These team members train volunteers from the community who have a desire to interact with hospice patients. These volunteers can offer companionship to patients. Some hospices will offer vigil volunteers who will sit with patients at EOL so that they are not alone when they die The coordinator may also arrange for massage therapists, pet therapy, music therapy, support for veterans, and even coordinate haircuts in the home. Some hospices arrange to honor hospice veterans in a special ceremony with their families. Volunteer veterans perform these ceremonies. I've attended several events, and they are special times for patients and their families. At times, local florists will donate flowers to patients and families. The hospice coordinator will arrange to distribute them to your patients, or you can pick some up at the office and deliver them yourself. The volunteer services offered vary with each hospice company.

I encourage you to take the time to get to know your team. I have thought of my hospice team as scaffolding that supports and stabilizes you. Remember, you are a valuable part of the hospice team, just like each team member. Working and collaborating well together is a wonderful thing in your hospice work.

THOUGHTS AND NOTES:

How has this knowledge about your hospice team made you aware of the support resources available to you? During your orientation, be sure to ask for visits with these team members or at least spend some time talking with them. Always remember that your team is your support system.

"Alone we can do so little; together we can do so much." - Helen Keller

There was something very special about Team 1007, my first hospice team. We were more than team members; we became good friends. We knew we had each other to celebrate the good times and always knew we had someone to lean on during tough times. Our HMD, Dr. Shariff, started having team lunches every other Friday (on payday) to have some downtime and enjoy each other's company. He found all the best restaurants in the area, and we enjoyed food and fun for about an hour on Fridays. This was the team I bonded with the most. To this day, I still keep in touch with some of them.

SUNSET MEMORY

CHAPTER 8

IDT AND RECERTIFICATIONS

IDT Meetings

IDT or Interdisciplinary Team meetings happen every two weeks, or "no less frequently than every fifteen calendar days," per the National Hospice and Palliative Care Organization (NHPCO). Generally, the HMD, RN case managers, social workers, chaplains, bereavement counselors, and maybe a volunteer coordinator are present at these meetings. There might also be a pharmacy representative attending. Each hospice team's routine will be different. During the meeting, your team discusses the plan of care for each of your patients and all the patients your RNCM colleagues have. You are responsible for giving updates or changes in your plan of care for your patients to the team since the last IDT meeting. Before your meeting, this information must also be documented in your patients' charts. Be sure to ask your nursing colleagues how to do this during orientation so you are prepared.

These meetings may last three to four hours, depending on how efficient your team is during discussions about each patient. It's important to be concise and to the point so you don't waste time. During an IDT meeting with a previous hospice team, each nurse was timed when giving report. We had a designated person to redirect us if we went off on a tangent. Getting off track is easy, so efficiency is vital during these meetings.

Before the COVID pandemic of 2020, team meetings used to be in person, and all of our team members met in one of the office conference rooms. During the pandemic, our team meetings turned into virtual meetings via Zoom or other video conferencing platforms which are Health Insurance Portability and Accountability Act (HIPAA) compliant. These video conferencing have continued since then in many hospice companies, mainly for convenience and as a time saver. Many teams have continued with Zoom meetings, and I have heard of others who have returned to in-person meetings. When you are done giving your report about your patients via Zoom, you are free to leave the meeting or stay on if you like. During orientation and a few months beyond, it would benefit you greatly if you stayed on and took the time to listen to the other nurses on how they give reports. If they have complex patients to discuss, it would be advantageous to listen to how problems are worked out as a team in case you have the same situation with your own patients. I've learned a lot just by listening and observing in IDT meetings.

Recertifications

Hospice is a Medicare benefit that is measured in benefit periods. At IDT meetings, your HMD will track upcoming recertifications, and your HMD or your clinical supervisor will notify you when recertifications (written documentation that the patient is still eligible for hospice) are due during IDT meetings.

On admission to hospice, a patient is given an initial certification by the patient's primary care provider and by the hospice attending physician. . Both providers will need to collaborate and agree that the patient is appropriate for hospice care and meets the Medicare criteria. This first benefit period is ninety days, and the second is ninety days.

About two to four weeks before the third benefit period starts, a face-to-face (F2F) visit is required with the hospice physician or nurse practitioner. Depending on how your hospice team conducts them, you may be asked to accompany the hospice physician or nurse practitioner during those F2F visits. I have been on many joint visits with our team's hospice physician or nurse practitioner. The knowledge of your patients, whether they are at home or in a facility, can help expedite these visits by showing them where the patient is and which family members or facility staff to talk to for pertinent information about your patient.

Your responsibility before the F2F visits is to write a recertification report using the Local Coverage Determination or LCD specific to your patient's hospice diagnosis as a guide. You can find this in the Hospice Quickflips© booklet, which your hospice will probably give you, or your clinical supervisor will provide a handout with this information. There are several LCDs, including cancer, ALS, dementia, etc. If a patient's condition does not fit in one of these categories, there is a "General Decline in Clinical Status" LCD to use. In this report, you will need to include specific details of decline, including weight loss, decreased arm circumference, decline in condition, and functional status. Other important information includes infections, hospitalizations, and falls, which show an additional decline in your patient's status. Essentially, you are proving that your patient is still eligible for hospice services for another benefit period.

During the F2F visit, you need to be ready with all the information you've gathered, as mentioned above, to give to your HMD or NP so they can include it in their report. You'll be able to discuss your patient's status and collaborate with your HMD/NP on the decline you have observed in the previous months.

Benefit periods will be sixty days long from now on for as long as the patient is in hospice. A F2F visit will be required, and you will need to write a recertification report two to four weeks before the end of each one.

Discharge From Hospice

Yes, believe it or not, patients can be discharged from hospice. When recertification is coming up for a patient, and you cannot provide enough evidence to show that your patient is hospice-appropriate, your team as a whole may conclude during the IDT meeting that your patient is no longer eligible for hospice services. Discharge planning should start as soon as possible. A discharge date will be decided on during the IDT meeting so you will know right away when it is. There should also be a discharge checklist for you and the team to follow. Make sure to ask your clinical supervisor for guidance when you do your first discharge since there are specific details you need to complete.

Other types of discharge from hospice include revocation (usually when the patient wants to continue curative measures), when the patient wants to transfer to another hospice, or when a patient moves out of the area of service from your hospice.

Here are some tips for reporting during IDT:

1. During your orientation, pay close attention to how your nurse colleagues give report during the IDT meetings. How does your HMD prefer the information to be presented? For example, one of my previous HMDs preferred the nurses to say the name, age and hospice diagnosis before we started giving report. Other HMDs did not require

this information. Be sure to follow the format of your hospice team's reporting, as each team has different ways to do it.

2. Explain in a short summary what has changed in each patient's status since the last IDT meeting.

3. Bring up any concerns or issues about your patients that require a discussion with the entire team. This may include any medication or symptom management issues, family dynamic or safety issues, patients you think are no longer appropriate for hospice services, patients moving to another location out of your service area, etc.

4. Be concise in giving reports so that the meetings are efficient and end on time.

5. If there are no new issues with your patient's condition or status, it's appropriate to say something like "Continue plan of care" or "Care managed well with the current plan of care." Again, use the words that your hospice team uses to convey this message.

THOUGHTS AND NOTES:

Now that you know that you are required to write recertification reports, take the time to ask your nurse colleagues about how they do this during orientation. Every nurse has a different way of doing these reports, so ask and learn from them. What questions do you have about this chapter?

"Heart is what separates the good from the great." - Michael Jordan

Before the 2020 COVID-19 pandemic, IDT meetings used to be in-person instead of online on Zoom. I looked forward to seeing my team members to chat, catch up before the meeting, and get hugs. I'm definitely a hugger. We celebrated everyone's birthdays with a card, a potluck (whatever people wanted to contribute), and a delicious dessert. Usually, the social workers would plan this, and I was more than happy to help them. I miss those days. Zoom meetings are convenient but cannot replace the bonding and camaraderie that in-person meetings provide. Your team may plan other events to get together, so be sure to attend those when possible.

SUNSET MEMORY

CHAPTER 9

HOME PATIENTS VERSUS FACILITY PATIENTS

Depending on how your hospice company is structured, you will either be on a team focusing on home patients, just facility or long-term patients, or a combination of the two. When I first started hospice work, our team primarily serviced long-term care facilities like care homes, nursing homes, retirement homes, assisted living facilities, etc. There are similarities between the two, but there are also definite differences.

Home Patients

Focus on teaching:
When your patient is at home, a lot of teaching needs to be done with the caregivers. They may be family members or paid caregivers who need instructions on caring for their loved ones or patients. Some family members have never cared for a sick loved one, so you will have to start from scratch and really get down to the basics. Even if you have paid caregivers, they may not have cared for a dying patient before, so you will need to give them a lot of instructions, too. As you can see, as a hospice nurse, you will be doing a lot of teaching and guiding. Be sure to give instructions clearly so families fully understand what you're teaching them. If they give you a blank stare or a "deer in the headlights" look, then you know you will have to repeat what you have instructed. If you notice during your visit that there is a change in your patient's condition, make sure to explain to family members what's happening and what to expect.

Affirm and instill confidence:
Keep teaching until you see they have confidence in themselves to do whatever you've taught them. If they are doing things well, I always sincerely tell them

that they are giving excellent care; saying "Good job!" or "You're doing great!" acknowledges their efforts and makes them feel good inside. They need to hear those words of affirmation. So don't hesitate to cheer them on. If family members have no caregiving experience at all, I allot more time to teach them or reinforce previous teaching.

What they learn from you will benefit them not only in the present moment but also in the future.

Family members will need instruction on comfort medications. Explain to them what each one is used for, when they are appropriate to be given, how much to give, and where to store them. Sometimes, when you admit a patient, the comfort meds are not needed right away. However, when a patient is nearing EOL, you will need to take more time to explain to family members and caregivers how to administer these meds. It might even be a good idea to draw up a few liquid meds like morphine and lorazepam in syringes just in case they need it overnight or on the weekend if it's coming up.

Family members need self-care too:
Caregiving is difficult and exhausting for families. Encourage family members to take turns and alternate caring for their loved one. This way, they can have rest time and not get worn out. If they don't have family help, you can ask your social worker to assist in finding paid caregivers. I've seen some patients who only have one family member, others who have many, and I've also seen patients who have no one.

Here are a few additional things to remember about home hospice patients:

- Call early on the day of their visit and tell them the approximate time of your visit. Be courteous and call if you're going to be late.

- As with all of your patients and families, take the time to really listen to them. You may discover insightful things about them if you take a few extra minutes to talk. This will strengthen your relationship with them and build their trust in you.

- Make sure they have enough meds at home before the weekend, especially before holidays and long weekends.

Facility Patients
When you are seeing patients in a facility, the focus is much different from

caring for home patients. The facilities include assisted living, memory care, nursing homes, care homes, and foster homes. Keep in mind that every facility you enter is a business. Each one has its own rules, routines, and regulations for caring for its residents. To them, you are considered a visitor or an outsider. So, to be successful in facilities, the one major thing to keep in mind is to provide good customer service and build good relationships with the staff on an ongoing basis. All of this takes time, so take the time to communicate with them. Your visits may be longer at first because you are trying to get to know everyone, and that's ok.

Good communication is vital for working well in facilities. Always introduce yourself when you enter a facility. Get to know the staff and their roles. Aim to be respectful of the facility's procedures.

Build trust:
A huge part of providing good customer service in facilities is building trust. The staff often view their residents as family members. When you come into a facility, the staff will be observing you to see if you are someone they can trust. And for the next few weeks and months, they will watch how you operate. Take this time to consistently show a friendly, caring attitude. When a staff member calls you about a problem, be sure to take care of it and answer any questions as quickly as you can. If you are busy at the moment, tell them a time when you can address their problem so they know you are going to take care of their needs. Make sure you call them back and follow through.

At my first hospice job, our team was the long-term care (LTC) team. We focused on working with patients primarily in facilities. It took quite a while for me to adjust to each facility on my caseload. Still, I just kept getting to know the staff, providing good care to their residents (what they call your patients), figuring out their procedures and routines, and communicating well with them. Essentially, my goal was to be an extension of their staff, the hospice expert. I focused on being a nurse they could rely on and depend on. After doing this week after week and month after month, I noticed that after a year, just about every facility I worked at started referring exclusively to our hospice company. My caseload skyrocketed.

I believe this was because the facility staff knew they could trust my care for their residents. I had established strong relationships by then, so they did not hesitate to refer their residents to our company.

But you would be wrong if you thought my numbers increased because of what I did exclusively. When facilities look at what your hospice company offers, they are not just looking at you, the hospice nurse; they are looking at your whole team. They look at your HMD, NPs, social workers, chaplains, and CNAs. We all had to work well together as a cohesive hospice team. The facility staff observed to see if the team gave their residents quality care. Make sure you are communicating important information and issues about your patients and facilities to your team, so everyone is aware and on the same page.

Build Good Relationships with Key People

There are some key staff you should be sure to get to know in your facilities.

- Meet the executive directors and administrative staff. When you first start visiting facilities, even during orientation, be sure to meet and introduce yourself to the executive directors or managers in your facilities. They will want to know who you are if you are coming into their community on a regular basis.

- Meet the care staff. These include the RNs, LPNs, medication technicians (med techs), and facility aides (each facility has different names for these aides, i.e., care partners). These are the people you will be coordinating care with regarding their residents at each visit, so get to know them well. I've made it a point to get to know the names of each one. It was a challenge to learn their names, but believe me, it will work to your best advantage if you do. If I couldn't remember their names, I wrote them down on paper until I did. I often needed help with something like turning a patient before doing wound care. Who did I call? The facility aides. If you have taken the time to know their names and build a relationship with them, they will readily assist you when you need an extra hand.

- Meet house doctors and nurse practitioners. Take the time to get to know the facility house doctors and nurse practitioners. These are the primary providers of the facilities and the ones who will refer residents to you. They will keep referring your hospice company if they have met you and know you are competent in caring for their patients.

At this point, you probably think there's so much to learn when seeing patients in facilities. And you're right, it is a lot. Don't rely on your memory in the beginning. Take lots of notes on what you observe about each facility. Ask the staff questions if you're not sure. You won't remember everything.

Be as thorough in your work as you can. You will discover what works and what doesn't through trial and error. That's why building trust and good relationships takes time. Give yourself grace when you make mistakes. Everyone has made their share of them. That's part of the learning process of this work.

Tips for Facilities

- Remember, your facilities have routines, schedules, and nuances. They all have their own way of doing things, like how to order meds and charting. Some facilities want you to word the medication orders you receive from your HMD/NPs in a certain way, so you need to follow through with that. Some facilities require you to do paper charting in their resident's physical chart, but others have their own computer charting, which you must learn how to use. Or the nursing staff may ask you to fax your note to their facility so they can put it in the patient's chart. You will need to know each facility's procedures to be compliant. Each facility will be surveyed by the State, which usually comes unannounced. Following the facility's procedures is important since you are from an outside company. If you are not doing things correctly, that facility may not continue to refer its residents to your hospice company. So, be sure to ask questions about their procedures and follow through with them.

- Be aware of mealtimes in facilities and avoid making visits at those times. The staff is usually too busy to give you updates on your patients. Since they are outside their rooms, the facility may not allow you to take vital signs and do physical assessments on your patients while sitting in the dining room with other residents around them. It's best to wait until after your patients are done eating their meals.

- Communicate with the nursing staff how your visit went and your plan of care for your patients. This is important to do at every visit so that the staff is aware of how your visit went and if there are any new orders you have written or faxed to them. The facility nurses have care plans for each resident too, which they discuss during their own facility meetings. The nurses may have some inside information you are unaware of, which would benefit your patients' care. That's why this coordination of care matters so much.

- Always wear your company badge when you enter a facility. This is for security purposes and to help the staff to identify you easily. Also, the

State might be in the building, and they want medical professionals to always wear their badges in-house.

- Be presentable and look professional when going to facilities. I always dressed in business casual attire since I knew I was stepping into a business. If you look professional, people will treat you as such. If your hospice company requires you to wear scrubs, then this will not be an option for you.

- Many facilities consider their communities (staff and residents) like family members. I mentioned this previously and wanted to emphasize this. During my hospice career, I have tried to focus on teamwork in each facility to be considered an extended part of the facility's "family," who is a hospice professional who manages caring for their terminally dying residents. But still being conscious to keep my emotional distance. There is a fine line to this. Just like home patients, tell the staff when you're available, from 8 a.m. to 5 p.m., so they don't call you during the night. You might get caught up in the drama of the facilities, but avoid doing this. Stay focused on caring for your patients and giving them the best possible care you can. As your hospice skills increase, the facility staff will look to you for guidance in caring for their dying residents. They are usually strong advocates for their residents who they have come to love and care for very much. They will tell you when things are not right or not going well with their residents, who they may consider their mom or dad or grandma or grandpa.

When I worked hard to build trust and provide good customer service to my facility staff members, I found it a joy to work with them. Even if there were problems, we worked them out the best we could. Once you have that teamwork in your facilities, consider it a victory and a success for you.

I also made observations about the different facilities I serviced. It is not what the building looks like on the outside that determines the quality of care given; it is the conscientious efforts of the staff.

Remember, your hospice company is a business. Another thing that you may not be conscious of as you begin this job is that the hospice company you work for is a business, too. Making sure you do your job to the best of your ability will help keep your company financially stable. That means striving to reach your company metrics, like addressing a patient's pain at every visit and keeping it 3/10 or less, doing your charting in a timely manner, etc. Also, make sure you use your time wisely during your patient visits by trying to see the recommended number of visits asked of you, which can be four to five or more, depending on your company. Sometimes this is possible, and sometimes it's not, depending on how complex your visits are. As you learn hospice, provide good care, and maintain strong relationships with facility staff, you also build your hospice company's reputation. You are the face of your hospice team. If you strive to do your best work, the staff will notice and keep referring patients to your company. This will help your company's census be at an optimal level.

State Survey

The department in your state that oversees facilities conducts surveys at every facility in your state to ensure compliance with their rules and regulations. To be in compliance, there are things you must do:

1. Chart your patient the way the facility requires of a visiting nurse. Ask the admin staff how to do this.

2. Communicate each patient's plan of care (POC) with nursing staff.

3. Make your visits brief and leave as soon as you can so you are not in the way of the staff. The State surveyors will come unannounced, so the facility must always be ready.

THOUGHTS AND NOTES:

This chapter was meant to give you a brief overview of what to expect before you visit home or facility patients. Do you have any thoughts or further questions? Be sure to ask the nurses who are orienting you or your mentor. Each hospice company has its own way of doing things, so be sure to ask for clarification so you know what to do.

"Nurses dispense comfort, compassion, and caring without even a prescription."
- Val Saintsbury

I was on the facility team during my first five years of hospice. We worked primarily in long-term care (LTC) facilities. At one particular facility, there was a med tech who was especially sweet and kind. I'd see her every morning, and she would greet me warmly and with a smile. She would always offer me a cup of coffee. Sometimes, I would accept, and other times, decline. One day, she said she made baklava and offered me a piece with a cup of coffee. How could I refuse? The baklava went perfectly well with my creamy coffee; it was not too sweet. I'll never forget her kindness.

SUNSET MEMORY

CHAPTER 10

MAKING YOUR VISITS

At the beginning of your orientation, you may be in meetings or doing learning modules on the computer to familiarize yourself with your hospice work.

Then, there will come a time when you will start going on visits with your team members and other nurse colleagues. You will learn many things about making visits by observing and asking questions. How you do visits may vary depending on the region of the country you live in. For example, the way you make visits will be somewhat different from an urban/city versus a rural/country area. Every RN case manager will do things a little differently, so watch closely how they do their work. Incorporate what you feel comfortable with into your own routine.

Closely watch how the nurses plan their visits. This visit planning is very important because RNCMs are required by Medicare to visit patients at least every fourteen days. You may want to use your calendar attached to your email or use a paper calendar to do this. If you are even a day late, that is considered to be out of compliance, and your company may be subject to fines by Medicare. So just be careful that your visits and assessments of your patients stay within the fourteen-day window. When you are on your own, your supervisor may ask you to use your email calendar to plan out your weeks so they can see who you will visit each day. Or, if you have a scheduler on your team, you will need to submit your patient visits a week ahead. Every hospice team is different, so follow your team's protocol.

Ask other nurses how they get their visits done during the week. When I first started planning my weeks, my supervisor advised me to do more visits at the beginning of my week so that I'd have time toward the end of the week to do my other documentation, like interdisciplinary team (IDT) notes and recertification reports. This also gives you a more open schedule to anticipate any urgent visits or if you have daily end-of-life (EOL) visits.

The following are basic steps for doing your nursing visits at the start of your day. Every day will not be the same as the previous day, so be flexible when the unexpected happens. You may need to readjust your schedule when urgent things come up.

1. As you look at your caseload, create a weekly schedule for all your patients. You will see some patients once a week and others two or three times a week. You can use your email calendar or a paper calendar and write each name on each day. From this, you can create a monthly schedule. Now you can see who you have to visit every day of the current month. When you have admissions, you will need to add those patients to your schedule, too.

2. At the end of the day, review who you are scheduled to see the next day. Be sure to get supplies you might need for your visits. The next morning, plan the route of your visits. You may want to work your way from the closest patient to your home to the farthest or work from the farthest to the closest patient. It helps to have this driving plan so you don't go in circles on the road, which is a waste of time and gas. Make sure you allow enough time for visits. I usually allow one-hour blocks of time at a patient's home and a little more at facilities. Be sure to plan for your lunch break. Even if it's ten to fifteen minutes, put it in there.

3. On the morning of your visits call patients and facilities to let them know when you will visit them. Some facilities prefer prior notice of your visit, and others don't. If a patient has an urgent need, you will need to see that patient first or sooner than later in your schedule. And if one of your patients is at EOL, you'll need to see that one first.

   As a courtesy, when you get behind in your time, call your patients or families to notify them that you will be later than scheduled and to let them know when to expect you to arrive.

4. Be aware of your surroundings once you arrive at your patient's home. Do you feel safe? Or is there something that makes you uneasy? Are

there dogs? If you feel unsafe, let your patient or family member know. Most patients are thoughtful and put their pets away before you visit. I have had patients put their dogs in their kennel or another room in their house so they don't disturb you during your visit. If you still feel unsafe, call and notify your clinical supervisor of what's happening. They may ask a social worker or other team member to accompany you.

5. Before you step into your patient's home or facility, take a moment to set aside any distractions from your previous patient's visit or anything from your personal life. Get yourself mentally ready to be fully present for this patient and their needs. Once you have entered the home, take the time to address any pressing matters or questions that the patient, family members, or paid caregivers have. This is the time to really listen to their needs or issues and take care of those things first. While you listen, be aware of your time because if you take too much time for one patient, you won't have enough for your other patients. Time management is an ongoing learning process. Give yourself grace when you first start seeing patients. Your caseload will be small in the beginning, so you can gradually take on more patients as you feel comfortable. I have a tendency to lose track of time, so I use my iWatch or iPhone and set a timer for forty-five minutes. When my timer goes off, I know I need to start wrapping up my visit.

6. Do your vital signs and assessment. See if any problems need addressing after doing this. You may find their blood pressure is low or high and need to intervene. Or they have a new wound you need to care for and teach the family or caretaker how to do it in your absence. Learn to assess pain thoroughly, noting location, description, and duration. Ask the questions, "What is your pain goal?" and "What makes the pain less, better, or worse." Patients and families will look to you as the hospice nurse to be an expert at providing good pain relief. They will look to you to quickly and effectively provide comfort to your patients. Often, it may take extra time to get patients to a comfortable place. It may not happen during your visit. But as long as you are working toward getting them relief, then that's the main thing. Keep learning about pain management. Your patients will thank you for it. Be sure to coordinate the care of your facility patients with the nurse on duty or the med tech. Give updates on your visit with them and address the problems they may have with your patients.

7. During your visit, ask yourself if you see anything that your patient, family members, or facility staff would benefit from your teaching. This might be about giving comfort medications, how to use durable medical equipment (DME), or what to look for in their loved ones when they see new symptoms. Or it could even be that you see something your patient or family members should be aware of. Letting them know of these things can help them anticipate what may happen in the future. Teaching is an important aspect of your visit for home patients and their families. The more information they have, the more confidence they will have in their ability to be prepared in a crisis situation.

8. I am a believer in charting at the bedside, so I usually take out my laptop shortly after I arrive at a patient's home or facility. If I can chart for even a minute or two during my visit, that will help me spend less time charting at the end of my day. I will go over more of the documentation in Chapter 11. Practice this now to get better at it, and it will benefit you in the long run.

9. Ideally, you will want to schedule your next visit with your patients or family members at the end of each visit, especially if their visit frequency increases or decreases. You may decide together on a particular day or days like Monday and Thursday or Tuesday and Friday, according to what works for your patient. If you do this consistently with each patient, you will have created your patient schedule for the next week. There are variations of this with different hospice companies, though. Especially if they utilize visit nurses besides the RNCM to make visits. In those cases, there will be a scheduler on the team to assign patients to visit nurses according to the RNCM's weekly schedule, which has been submitted. When you do facility visits, you may want to designate certain days to see your patients. The staff will notice your routine as you communicate with them.

10. After you visit with facility patients, be sure to call your patients' main contact person to whom you are to give updates. You'll need to find out who this person is at admission. It could be their power of attorney (POA), designated health care representative, a close family member, or friends. This will give them an opportunity to share their concerns or ask you questions. Be consistent in calling this contact person for updates after every visit if they are not present during your visits. Believe me, they want to know what's going on with their loved one, especially if there are major changes in their condition.

Remember Your Role as a Nurse Guide

As you learn more about how to do this hospice nursing work, be careful to keep your role as a guide for your patients and their families. Are you familiar with the phrase, "They don't know what they don't know"? For patients and families, hospice is a dark road. You are the one who holds the lamp and will help them navigate this unknown path. It may be a very scary road to travel, so give them a picture of what lies ahead. Prepare them. How can they be ready? Always ask yourself, what do my patients and family need right now? You don't want to give too much information too soon. Being in hospice is overwhelming in itself. Yes, it is your responsibility to tell them what to anticipate, but ultimately, you should honor your patient's choice. We need to be careful not to push our biases on their journey to their end.

Here is a case in point. I had a patient who had refused to schedule morphine because he did not want to be "drugged up." Some other patients would agree with scheduling meds to stay comfortable, but not John. And guess what his reasoning was? He had a daughter who had died of a drug overdose, and he did not want to die that way. So, when I suggested it, and he said no, I did not push the issue. The best thing for me to do was to respect his wishes, collaborate with my HMD, and try other ways to manage his pain.

More About Safety

You can never be too cautious before entering a patient's home. The key is to be aware of what's happening around you so you can protect yourself. In all my years of hospice, I can only remember two or three times when I felt unsafe. I remember doing an admission for a young man who was a drug addict and lived in a "drug house." Before visiting, I talked with our HMD, and she asked me if I felt okay doing the admission. I told her I would not go into the home if I didn't feel safe. I was apprehensive at first, but when I stepped into the house, I did not feel like I was in danger. If I had, I would have gotten in my car and driven away. We all have our sixth sense or intuition. For the sake of your safety, you need to act on your gut instinct when you feel like you are in a dangerous situation.

The following visits are different types of visits you may need to make in your hospice work. I've described what needs to be done for each one.

Admission Visits

Some hospice companies have admission nurses who do these visits exclusively. But even if you have admission nurses on your team, there may be too many for them to handle on any given day. For this reason, it is essential that you learn how to do admission visits. Other hospice companies do not have admission nurses, so the task falls on you as the RN case manager. In that case, doing admissions will be something you need to learn and master.

When doing an admission visit, you need to ask yourself these two important questions.

1. "What medical information makes this patient hospice appropriate?"
2. From my assessment, do I think this person has less than six months to live?

In your charting, you will have to paint a picture of why this patient is hospice appropriate. There are Medicare guidelines to abide by and criteria to be met to admit a patient to hospice services. You may be communicating with your HMD to figure this out, especially if there is not much evidence for hospice eligibility. The referral for hospice generally comes from the patient's primary physician. Most of the time, hospice services are very appropriate, but sometimes they are not. There are instances when our HMD has notified the primary physician that their patient did not qualify for hospice and will need to wait for a further decline in their patient's status.

During the admission visit, you may meet with the patient's POA and maybe some family members who live nearby. It is ideal if your social worker is present to assist with the admission so that both of you can hear the patient's medical history explained by the patient and family at the same time. The social worker will describe hospice services and the scope of care to the patient, POA, and family. If there are any questions, they are free to ask them for clarification. If the patient is agreeable to hospice services, then consent forms will be signed at that time. If the patient is not able to do so, then the POA will sign the forms. During this discussion, we will ask if the patient has a Portable Orders for Life-Sustaining Treatment (POLST) form, which shows their wishes for medical treatment. This form is signed by the patient and by the team's HMD. I've worked at hospice companies that do admissions in a different way, so be sure to do an admission during your orientation.

After this discussion, you will need to do VS and assessment and address any new problems or manage symptoms. You will also need to give instructions for all the comfort medications ordered at the time of admission. You may pick up these meds from the pharmacy before going home. In a facility, the comfort meds are ordered from their designated pharmacy, and they will send them to the facility. Again, there may be variations to this according to your hospice company.

There is a hospice handbook you'll give to the patient and family and may need to give to the hospice facility staff as well. The home patients will be given a patient education folder with med instructional forms and other forms to write PRN (as needed) pain meds given to the patient. During your visit, you will also need to determine what durable medical equipment (DME), such as a hospital bed, bedside commode, oxygen concentrator, etc., your patient needs. You will then ask your office hospice staff for these items. If admitting a facility patient, the nurse will tell you what DME is needed.

As you can see, admission visits are longer than routine visits because many things need to be in place before admitting a patient. The average admission visit may take about an hour for uncomplicated cases. For patients with more complex cases, your visit may turn out to be two to three hours. The charting will also take much longer than the routine visits, which could be another one to two hours or more, depending on the patient.

End-of-life Visits

End-of-life (EOL) visits start when a patient begins to rapidly decline and transition to the end-of-life. Daily visits are required at this time to closely monitor and manage your patient's symptoms. Examples of this EOL decline include when the patient stops eating or drinking or when they have less verbal response or have a blank stare, and sleep time increases dramatically. When you see a sharp or steady decline like this, you may need to warn your families that you think this may be the start of their loved one's transition to end-of-life.

In the beginning, you may not see this, but as your experience increases over time, you'll recognize your patient's physical signs that their end is near. During this time, you will be doing daily visits to manage symptoms regarding pain, trouble breathing, anxiety, agitation, etc. This is also the time you will prepare the family for their loved one's end-of-life. These visits can be intense, and you will need more time to manage symptoms and to be present during this stressful time for families or friends. Be sure to allow for extra time for these visits.

During your EOL visits, you will need to make sure the patient and family have chosen a funeral home. If it is not already indicated on your patient's chart, you can provide a list of funeral homes from which they can choose. Usually, the social worker will have this list, or you can keep a copy in your folder so that you can give it to your family when it is time. The family should do this before their loved one dies. Trying to decide on a funeral home can be a nightmare when they're already dealing with their grief and sadness. I always explain it to them this way, and the family usually agrees. They will talk about it together and come to a decision. This will put their mind at ease as well since it's one less thing to worry about when their loved one dies. Sometimes, the family has put off this decision while their loved one has been in hospice care until this moment because of denial. It's ok for the family to do this since the thought of their loved one dying is too traumatic for them to think about. When they are ready, they will let you know. But when there's no more time to put it off, warn them that they need to make a decision.

When a patient's end is imminent, I warn the family that the time of their loved one's end is near. I encourage them to notify other family members, especially the ones out of state, so that they have the opportunity to visit and say their last goodbyes.

This would be a good time to ask the family if they want the hospice chaplain to visit. If so, you can request this. If the family prefers their loved one's minister to come and give last rites or pray over them, they will usually make that call. In instances when the family asks for clergy from a certain religion or denomination, like a Catholic priest, your hospice team's chaplain can arrange for that.

Always take full VS as part of your assessment when doing EOL visits. Vital signs can give clues as to the nearness of your patient's end. Having a fever is very common. Their heart rate may be elevated, over 100 and in the 120s. This is an indication of dehydration when the heart needs to pump harder to circulate blood all over the body. Their BP might be decreasing, which is a good indication of the end being imminent. It is important to make sure your patient has an adequate supply of comfort medications they need in the home or facility, especially before the weekend. You surely don't want to run out of meds on a Sunday when most pharmacies are closed.

During this time, try to give guidance to the family about what to expect. Refer them to the hospice handbook given to them at admission. It has valuable information about the dying process. Also, give them the booklet Gone From My Sight, written by Barbara Karnes, RN, which explains the phases of decline. Your hospice company will have a supply of this in the office, which you can give to families. Sometimes, this little booklet may be given at admission, depending on your hospice team's procedure. If the family needs one, this is the time to give it to them to prepare them for what's ahead.

Because caring for a loved one at the end-of-life is intense, I recommend that the family take rest breaks and alternate their times of care so they don't get worn out. Offer words of affirmation and encouragement to the family while caring for their loved one. Be there to support the family. Your presence is so needed at this time.

The Most Asked Question

While you are caring for your patients, you will be asked, "How long does my (loved one) have left to live?" From my experience, this question is most asked by family members. This question is often asked during or shortly after hospice admission. They ask so that they can plan for the next few days and weeks. They want to determine how long to stay. How long can they get off work? Do they need to take time through the Family and Medical Leave Act (FMLA) to care for their loved one? I explain my "educated" prognosis the way I learned it from a former HMD.

When a family member asks me to give a prognosis for their loved one, I explain it in three time frames:

1. **Hours to days:** If a patient appears imminent and at EOL, I will tell the family the prognosis is hours to days. The signs I look for are a patient being unresponsive, mouth breathing, no more eating food or drinking fluids, breathing patterns changing, etc., depending on how long their loved one wants to hold on. I learned early on not to underestimate the will to live. If the patient appears to be imminently dying but is waiting for a family member or close friend to come and say their goodbyes, they will hold on until that family member has arrived. And once their family member or friend comes, they will let go and die shortly afterward. I have seen this happen time and time again.

2. **Days to weeks:** If a patient is starting to physically decline and requires more symptom management for pain or agitation, falling more, or has worsening wounds, I will usually tell them their loved one has

days to weeks. Patients could even go through a sharp decline and die suddenly. This is what I tell families who have loved ones with a cardiac or respiratory diagnosis like congestive heart failure (CHF), third-degree block, COPD, pulmonary fibrosis, etc. I give them this warning so they are not surprised when sudden death happens. Or a patient might rally and have a really good day, and then the rapid decline comes. That is very common.

3. **Weeks to months:** When a patient is ambulating independently, able to feed themselves, and doing most of their activities of daily living (ADLs) with little or no active symptom management, then I will tell the family I think their loved one has weeks to months to live. After receiving regular visits and close monitoring from the hospice team, some patients' health status may improve. Some even thrive to the point of needing to be discharged from hospice services.

When you have chosen which time frame you think is most appropriate, always tell the family why you have come to that conclusion. What signs and symptoms did you see that have led you to believe how long a person has left to live? I usually give a recap of what has been happening to the patient, their decline, any symptoms that need to be managed, and where the patient is at that moment. This helps the family think through all the details and understand where their loved one is at that time. Then, I will tell them what time frame I think the patient is in.

I have used this method to tell families my "best" educated guess because I don't have a crystal ball, and I am not God. The family members understand that I will not be 100 percent correct. Once, I made the mistake of telling a family member that I thought their loved one had two or three days left to live, and that patient ended up living a whole week longer than I predicted. So, my point is that it is better to use the time frame method when giving a prognosis. It's a safe way to explain things to families and, of course, is less embarrassing for you.

You may be thinking, "Me, give a prognosis? Only doctors do that." I used to be intimidated by this question, too, but as I gained more hospice experience and used the time frame method, I became more comfortable explaining prognosis to families. This skill will take time for you to get used to, but as you do it more often, you will master it.

Death Visits

For a Home Patient

When your patient dies on your day shift and the family calls your team's hospice number, you will be asked to do the pronouncement visit. Some hospice companies require their nurses to do death visits; for others, it may be optional, depending on what the family wants. I have experienced both. I prefer doing death visits because you can be present with the family and provide comfort and closure while you are there. You have built relationships with your family members and facility staff, and being there at the end, to me, is an essential part of hospice nursing. Your presence in their grief means a lot, so take the time to be with the family during their loss.

During death visits, I offer my condolences to the family and give hugs (if the family members are huggers). They will usually tell me how their loved one died, whether witnessed or alone. The main thing I'm hoping to hear is that their loved one died peacefully. Then, I will take out my stethoscope and examine the patient to assess if they have a pulse or respiration. I do this by listening for a heartbeat with my stethoscope and then placing my hand on their chest to watch for a rise and fall in their breathing.

The family wants confirmation of their loved one's death. When you tell the family there is no heartbeat or respirations, they have your official verification. I will then call their primary physician's office and notify them, notify the HMD, and let the hospice office staff know the time of death (TOD). Technically, the time of death is the time when you pronounce it. But there are times when the family wants the time of death to be when they saw the last breath or discovered that the patient died. If that happens, use the family's time of death. In the state that I work in, I can use the family's time of death. But this may vary and will depend on the state law where you work. Next, I will call the funeral home of the patient or family's choice and give them all the information they need, including the patient's name, date of birth, address, TOD, and the next of kin or POA contact information.

The funeral home will also ask which physician will sign the death certificate. It is usually the patient's primary physician; if unable to do so, your HMD will probably sign it. On average, a funeral home usually takes one to two hours to pick up the patient. You might ask if the family needs more time with their loved one. If not, then let the funeral home know they can come.

If the family needs more time, then let the funeral home know and ask the family to call the funeral home when they are ready for their loved one to be picked up.

Next, you will need to give instructions on how to dispose of controlled meds/narcotics. Some hospice teams require the hospice nurses to appropriately dispose of the narcotic or controlled meds together with the family, so find out what your team's protocol is. Afterward, tell the family that a bereavement counselor will contact them in about four weeks to follow up on their grieving process and provide support.

One thing the family may ask for is postmortem care, in which case you would help the family give their loved one a complete bed bath. You can also offer this postmortem care yourself. This is one of the most sacred tasks you will do as a hospice nurse. As you assist the family in bathing their loved one, putting on a special outfit, and making their loved one presentable, you are creating a special memory with the family that they will remember forever.

For a Facility Patient

When you do a death visit for a facility patient, the family may or may not be there, but again, offer your condolences to the family members who are present. The facility staff will also be grieving at that time, so offer your condolences to them. Do your pronouncement and give the nurse on duty the time of death. Call and notify the funeral home and give them the pertinent information. The facility has its own protocol for wasting the patient's narcotic meds, so you don't have to worry about that. If the family is present, notify them of the bereavement counselor's call in about four weeks to provide grief support. The family or facility staff may also ask for your assistance in doing postmortem care at that time, so go ahead and graciously do this task. This sacred act of kindness is a gift you give to families and the facility staff.

Hospice Levels of Care

In hospice, there are four different levels of care. These are routine care, continuous care, general inpatient care (GIP), and respite care. The visits you do daily are considered routine care. Continuous care is provided around the clock by your hospice company in-home or in the facility. GIP care may be provided in a hospital or hospice facility. Respite care allows family caregivers a break in caring for their loved ones. A patient is transferred to a Medicare-certified inpatient facility for this kind of care. There are hospice requirements for each level of care. You will be required to make a certain number of nursing visits while your patient is under any of these levels of care other than routine care.

Continuous Care Visits

Sometimes, your patient's symptoms, like acute pain or agitation, may need closer monitoring. You have talked with your HMD and have come up with a plan of care for managing their pain, but you hesitate to leave them alone. Continuous care for their patients might be a good option for these patients. Not all hospice companies offer this, but if your company does, take full advantage of this service as it could provide a substantial level of support to your patient, their family members, and facility staff if they reside in a facility for symptoms like uncontrolled pain or agitation. The first hospice company I worked for offered this care in homes and facilities.

The National Hospice and Palliative Care Organization (NHPCO) describes continuous care as "Predominantly nursing care, covered for at least eight hours and up to twenty-four hours." I explained to families that a hospice continuous care staff would help manage their loved one's symptoms, whether it was pain or agitation. My first hospice company tried to schedule staff to cover twenty-four hours, but there were some hours that the family needed to cover when staffing was not available. The way your hospice company provides continuous care will be different, or this option may not even be offered in your company.

While your patient is receiving continuous care, you must make a visit daily to assess how well their pain or agitation is being managed and collaborate with your HMD to make any necessary changes. Once the acute symptom is managed well, the continuous care will be discontinued.

GIP Visits

These visits are also daily ones. These patients may be placed in the hospital or in a hospice inpatient unit where care is provided twenty-four hours a day. When you make your visit, you will need to assess your patient's uncontrolled symptoms like pain or anxiety/agitation. If changes need to be made, notify your HMD for new orders. This care is also designed to be short-term to closely manage acute symptoms that the family may have difficulty managing at home. Once the symptoms are under control, your patient will be transported back home.

Respite Care Visits

When you see family members beginning to experience caregiver burnout, respite care can be offered for up to five days. Your patient will be transferred to a Medicare-certified facility for this care. When your patient is transferred to a facility for respite care, make sure to visit the facility on the day of the transfer to assess if they are settling in well and communicate and coordinate care with the facility staff. You will need to make another visit during the five-day period or possibly more if there are any issues you need to take care of with the staff.

Inpatient Hospice Facility Visits

Some hospice companies have an inpatient facility for their hospice patients for end-of-life symptoms or when the family is willing to privately pay for their loved ones to receive care there. This would depend on room availability at the time. If your company has one, and your patient transfers from home to an inpatient facility, you will still need to make your routine visits there.

On-call Visits

Once you have had enough experience under your belt, your supervisor may ask you to pick up some on-call hours or days. I believe I wasn't asked to do this until I had completed a year of hospice. It is usually the weekend or the evening hours that are needed for on-call. Your team will have after-hours or on-call nurses who come on duty after 5 p.m. When they go on vacation or are unavailable, these on-call hours/days will cover those that are open. If you have been on call, it's essentially triage work. You will be addressing patients' urgent problems or issues.

You will receive calls from patients or family members with questions, concerns, or an urgent need. If the problem is too much to solve over the phone, you will need to visit. Sometimes, it's a symptom management problem or maybe a death visit. Since hospice services are offered twenty-four-seven, doing on-call work is essential to a hospice team. You never know when there is an urgent need.

When patients or family members call, they are trying to solve some issue and need your advice on what to do. They may be anxious or panicked about a problem. Having a calm and steady voice when you talk to them is vital. Allow them to talk and find out what their concerns are. Then, give options and solutions for their problems. If a medication needs to be adjusted, you will need to contact your HMD on duty,

Sometimes, I've gotten calls from family members who just need reassurance that what they are doing for their loved one is correct. If it is, I affirm them. If not, I give them instructions. Other times, family members have called for a particular problem requiring a visit, but I see a completely different problem once I get there. So, just be ready for the unexpected when you do on-call visits. It is wise to keep an adequate stock of supplies in your nurse's box in your car in case you need to do wound care, change a Foley, problem-shoot a patient-controlled analgesia (PCA) line, etc. If you don't have these essential supplies, you will have to spend extra time going to the office to pick up what you need. Feel free to ask your nurse colleagues what they keep in a nursing supply box in their car for emergencies.

Remember This:
From the orientation of my first hospice company, I distinctly remember something one of our administrative doctors, Dr. Cameron Muir, said in a video when he talked about patient/family interaction. He said, "This is NOT a dress rehearsal; it's the real thing." Whatever you do or say will be forever etched in the minds of your patients' families long after their loved ones have passed away. You will have a huge impact on them. He encouraged us to do our jobs well because we often don't get a second chance to do it right.

Patients and families will know and feel it when you do your best work for their loved one. Things may not go perfectly. You will make mistakes, and that's okay. Learn from them and go on. Whatever you go through in the future, you have the experience to know what to do when those situations arise again.

I say this because you are just starting in hospice. I want to encourage you to do your best work, give the best care you possibly can, and give yourself grace when things don't go exactly the way you want them to. Remember that what you did during your visits was enough, and you will not be perfect in every situation and with every patient. And that is ok. Cherish the good memories and learn from the bad ones.

THOUGHTS AND NOTES:

After you've made some visits with your nurse colleagues in orientation, you will begin to understand what is required for different kinds of visits. Be sure to ask questions during your visits if you need clarification. If you are thinking of any questions now, write them down here and ask them later.

"To do what nobody else will do, a way that nobody else can do, in spite of all we go through; that is to be a nurse." - Rawasi Williams

I remember when my colleagues and I celebrated a patient's birthday. He was a veteran in his nineties. Arion, our chaplain, and Kathleen, our social worker, were present. I brought a chocolate cake I made but forgot to bring plates and napkins. I scrounged around in his kitchen for paper towels or napkins but couldn't find any. I spied some coffee filters on the counter, and we ended up using those to eat our chocolate cake. It was a funny and memorable time with our patient.

SUNSET MEMORY

CHAPTER 11

HANDLING DIFFICULT FAMILIES

It is highly likely that you will have some patients with difficult and dysfunctional family dynamics on your caseload.

When a patient is in hospice care, it is essential that family members work together to care for their loved one. Unfortunately, we do not live in a perfect world, and that does not always happen. I have had the pleasure of knowing families who get along well and other families who have strained relationships.

Fortunately, you will have the support of your social workers, who can help you navigate family conflicts and unhealthy behaviors along the way. Reach out to them when you are having difficulty with family members. Two is better than one in this case. Also, when you meet during interdisciplinary team (IDT) meetings (discussed in Chapter 8), be sure to discuss the challenges you face with these patients' family members. During your collaboration, your team may come up with ways to cope with and manage sensitive situations you haven't thought of.

The point is, you are not alone, so don't try to do it alone. It will wear you out.

When you start to feel like you are spending a lot more time at a patient's home with overwhelming family issues or you see family dynamic problems that are beginning to take a lot of your time and energy, ask for help right away. I have asked our social workers to help intervene in these cases. You can ask them to make more frequent visits and determine their family needs. Is it caregiving-related? Or is a family member causing chaos? Is a family feeling overwhelmed and anxious and just needs more time to talk with a hospice team member? It could be a variety of reasons. But whatever it is, I'll say it again: don't do it alone. Get to know your social workers early on. They can be your best support in your daily work.

It's also good to know that some family issues are deeply rooted in years of dysfunction. It is not your responsibility to change or improve family relationships. Sometimes, you need to allow families to work out their problems and let them know that the hospice team is there to support their decisions.

Ultimately, your role as a hospice nurse is to help families concentrate on caring well for their loved ones in their last days of life, however chaotic their family dynamics may be. Focus on how they can help make the end for their loved one as peaceful and comfortable as possible. Usually, a power of attorney (POA) is the most level-headed or pragmatic one in the family and will advocate for this. That's probably why their loved one chose them to make sure their wishes were honored and followed through.

Also, with these challenging cases, I've told my clinical supervisor about these families right away so that a plan can be put in place. Perhaps a family meeting with your HMD, social worker, and you are what's needed to coordinate care and answer questions that the family has so that all of you can come to an agreement on a reasonable plan of care for your patient.

At the beginning of your hospice work, it can get frustrating if things aren't going smoothly with families. I have had many instances when I had to do some kind of conflict resolution. At first, it was uncomfortable. But with the help of my social workers and other team members, by observing them, I learned the words to say and how to deal with families in difficult situations. With time and more experience, your comfort level will increase. It may seem hard to believe now, but you will develop a thicker skin and be able to handle these challenges more effectively.

The ultimate goal of family conflict resolution is to create understanding among family members. A disagreement or argument within the family may have occurred years ago and has not been resolved since. Allowing families to communicate with each other, even though it creates a conflict, can actually be beneficial to all in starting the healing process. I have seen that happen many times. Relationships may not greatly improve but I've observed that most families will try to cooperate for the sake of their loved one.

THOUGHTS AND NOTES:

How do you handle conflict? What is your comfort level with conflict? These questions are to create awareness of your past experience. Dealing effectively with conflicts and family problems is a skill you will learn in this work.

During orientation, you may encounter tough family problems. Watch and observe how your team members handle these issues. Ask your social workers how they handle difficult family problems. Be aware of your comfort level with conflicts and resolving them.

Take a moment to write your thoughts. The good thing about family conflicts in your work is that you're not alone. Your team will do what they can to support you. Learn from them.

"Nurses are the calm in the chaos, the hope in the despair, and the light in the darkness." - Unknown

Mino was my hospice nurse buddy. If I needed help with something I couldn't quite do right, she was always willing to help. Or if I just needed to talk things through or commiserate and laugh about our days' battles, she was my listening ear. For all those times, Mino, thank you!

SUNSET MEMORY

CHAPTER 12

MANAGING CHARTING AND DOCUMENTATION

Charting is a major part of your work and can be challenging to manage. It will take up a lot of your time as a case manager, so making adequate time for charting is very important.

There are a variety of ways to approach and complete your charting. Some nurses focus on making their visits first and then charting after seeing all their patients. Others chart while they are at their patient's home. Or nurses chart in their cars or other places like the library or at a coffee shop. I know a nurse who charted in libraries between visits just to get something done. I have charted in all these different ways and have come to one conclusion. If I charted something during my visits or shortly after, I would most likely be able to finish my charting at the end of the day or early evening. If I waited until I got home, took care of my family, and finished some house cleaning, I would be too tired to finish all my charting.

I highly recommend learning the skill of charting as you do your visits during the day. Incorporate five to ten minutes during or shortly after your visits for charting time. I set my cell phone timer for five minutes on busy days and just did speed charting. You would be surprised how much you can chart in five minutes. For example, if I charted on my four patients during their visits for even five minutes, I would have twenty minutes less to chart in the evening.

Some nurses feel awkward getting out their laptops during their visits and charting while talking to their patients and family members. I totally understand that. It can seem impersonal. But I have found a way to chart during a visit that works for me. At the beginning of my visit, I take the time to listen to the main problems or issues my patient is going through and needs help with. During that time, I'll listen and may write notes on my daily visit form. (I created this form on my own and have included it at the end of Chapter 16.) Once they are done explaining their needs, I open my laptop, take their vital signs, and do my assessment. When I'm done with that, I take my laptop and start charting something—anything. I chart quickly and succinctly for about a minute or two so that I have something done.

Believe me, it feels good to see even partial charting completed when I sit down later in my day to do my documentation. It's like when you see your primary doctor. At some point during your visit, your doctor will be charting on their computer about you. During your visit, you are doing the same thing for your patients. If family members have questions, I answer them during this time. If you can multitask and your family member is chatty and talks a lot, you can chart more, so it depends on the family. If you do this consistently during every visit, you will train yourself to chart and train the patient and family to know this is a normal part of your visit. It's a win-win situation.

If you are having difficulty charting on time, talk to your supervisor. The goal is to complete your charting on the evening of your visits. Find out what your hospice company's expectation of charting is. Having a small caseload is ideal in the beginning so that you can manage your visits and charting time well. I started off with five to six patients, and then, as I could manage those, my supervisor gradually increased my caseload.

As you are learning how to do hospice nursing, there are going to be days that you are just way too busy to chart during or shortly after your visits. Some visits may turn out longer than anticipated, and nothing seems to go as planned. Yes, these stressful and chaotic days will happen, and when they do, please don't be too hard on yourself. Try to find a window of opportunity in your day to chart something, even for five to ten minutes. Learn from these kinds of days and go on.

I recommend that you make it a goal to finish your visits by 3 or 4 p.m. That way, you will give yourself time to chart and complete a substantial amount. Being concise in your charting will also reduce your overall charting time. I usually prioritized inputting all new medication orders. It's important to get those in first and finish charting on those patients. That way, the on-call night nurse has access to those new orders if the family or facility staff calls about any concerns or issues overnight.

Look back at the end of the day and see how you could have done things better. If you can improve your process or the way you do things, then go ahead and make those adjustments. If it was a crazy day, give yourself grace and know tomorrow will be different. Hopefully, it will be a lighter, more manageable day.

The honest reality of hospice nursing is that your charting will spill over into your evenings. How much it spills will depend on you. The more you chart during work hours, the less you need to chart when you get home. I strongly suggest that you practice good time management during your visits so that you have time to finish your charting. Take care of the problems at hand and try not to linger too long at a patient's home or facility.

If you have a family, make this a priority and chart as much as you can during the day. Do it for the love of your family. Do it so you can focus your time on them when you go home. Also, make time for yourself to rest and recover. My family and rest time were huge motivators for charting during my day. If you are single, make it a priority to do as much charting as possible during your workday so you can have that rest time, too. Hospice work can be exhausting, so be good to yourself and keep improving your time management.

Tips for Documentation:

- Chart the decline of your patient.

- Make it a priority to get weights and mid-arm circumference (MAC) at the start of each month and include them in your recertification reports. Make sure to use the same arm every month. Ask your nurse colleagues how they do their MACs. Each hospice company has its own procedure.

- Keep track of significant events during the certification period, even between IDTs, like falls, infections, hospitalizations, and significant decline. I talked about this previously in the IDT Chapter 8. I knew a nurse who was very organized and documented in her own notebook when all these significant events happened for each patient. It was just a little note so she could use that information in her recertification report.

Part of your charting will include a plan of care (POC). We nurses know all about this. Your patient's POC is initiated during the admission visit. If problems come up with your patient, like a new wound or the need to place a Foley, you will need to add this to your patient's POC. Your plan of care is your patient's problem list that you address when you make your visits. These care plans will guide your visits so you know what to focus on. If another nurse sees your patients, a quick overview of your patient's POC will guide that nurse and help them determine what problems to address. These care plans should be updated when any changes are made. Your clinical supervisor will ask that your POC goals be specific to the needs of your patients. Be sure to ask your nurse colleagues how to do this during orientation. When your hospice company gets surveyed, the POC for each patient will be examined, so it is very important to keep track of it.

THOUGHTS AND NOTES:

How will you plan to do your hospice charting? Ask your nurse colleagues how they do theirs. Observe the pros and cons of each one. Which methods have you chosen to use? How will you make it work for you?

"The efficiency of a person's work is directly proportional to the intensity of his interest in excellence." - Tom DeMarco

I am a detailed person by nature, and I found that this did not work to my advantage when charting. I wanted to include every little detail of my visit. That wasn't really necessary. When I read other nurses' notes, which were briefer and more concise and, in essence, said the same thing I would've said in fewer words, I knew I had to change my approach to charting. When I did that, I was able to finish charting sooner and have more downtime for myself. That felt so good!

SUNSET MEMORY

CHAPTER 13

FIND WAYS TO PROCESS YOUR GRIEF WORK

Grief work and healing are not just for your patients and families but also for you.

As you see patients, you may soon become attached to them. They may be here one day; the next day or week, they're gone. As a hospice nurse, part of your job is going through this loss, too. It's like a cycle of grief, as a former bereavement counselor colleague called it.

As you help your patients and family members go through the dying process, part of your work is also to recognize that you need to do your own grief work. It's hard losing patients and seeing them die, and that loss will affect you emotionally. As you know, it is not easy to go through the grieving process. Some patients will mean more to you than others, so their loss will impact you more. I advise you not to bottle up or ignore these painful feelings of sadness. Take the time to work through this grief.

I remember in my early years of hospice when I had multiple deaths in a week. I have had up to three patients die in one week. That felt brutal. I felt a deep sadness as I was reeling from the grief. It was hard to care for the rest of my patients while thinking of the ones I'd lost. That's one of the hardest things to go through as a hospice nurse: multiple losses in a short span of time. It's hard to accept the loss at first because you've developed a bond with your patients and their families. When it was unbearable, I would call our bereavement counselor to talk. She would say I needed to take some time to work out my sadness and feelings of loss. If I didn't take the time to work these emotions out, I would have a continued sense of uneasiness, like I had unfinished business. When you feel this way, don't sweep your feelings under the rug or ignore them. It is a cue that you have some grief work to do. This emotional care is an essential part of hospice nursing, which will help you thrive in this work if you take the time to do it.

You might be tempted to skip this part of your work, but please don't.

In hospice, if you continue your work without addressing your emotions from previous patients who died, you may feel a heaviness, like a burden of sadness you carry around with you. I have felt this way before. Through the help of my teammates, I learned how to work through my grief.

So how do you do this grief "processing"? Here are several ways you can do it:

1. **Journaling:** Take five to ten minutes, or more, at the end of your day to write down the emotions you are feeling going through a particular loss. Putting thoughts down on paper may clarify the mixed-up emotions you are feeling at the time. You can journal in the little notebook I mentioned earlier (the one you use for daily notes) or use a bigger journal. I have a separate journal simply because I want more space to write. And sometimes, when I'm tired, I journal on my mini-iPad. Those days, I find it faster to type than write. However, if you want to journal, do what's best for you. Whatever you choose, just get it out of your head.

2. **Talking it out:** Another option is to talk about your loss to someone. The social workers, bereavement counselors, and chaplains are good people to reach out to. They are generally good listeners who can offer tools to help you verbalize and work through your loss. I found they had perspectives I had never considered or ways to cope with my sadness. Sometimes, they helped me clarify my confusion over a difficult case. I have learned so much from those with many years of hospice experience under their belts.

3. **Doing something active:** Having a physical outlet can help you work things through in your mind and release the stress and tension of losing a patient. You might choose to go for a walk, bike ride, or work out at the gym. Or you might want to try being creative and make something with your hands. This could be doing crafts, trying a new recipe, or baking your favorite cookies. I've enjoyed crocheting after work because it's mindless, it keeps my hands busy, and I can do it purely for fun.

On really tough days, the one thing I need most when I come home is hugs. I am so thankful when I get hugs from my family. It is a stress reliever, and it's nice to get a little TLC when you've given so much during your workday.

4. **Counseling:** One thing that has really helped me in my grief work is professional counseling. At my first hospice job, I used our company's Employee Assistance Program (EAP) as often as I could. Part of that EAP included a counseling service. It was a work benefit, so no out-of-pocket cost to me. I could speak to a counselor twenty-four hours a day and discuss any dilemma I was going through. This included anything personal or work-related. It was a valuable resource for me. Whenever I called, I would get a new counselor to talk with. The conversations usually lasted about fifteen to twenty minutes. Each counselor was very supportive and knowledgeable in helping me through any problem I struggled with during my workday. They were always able to help me make sense of what I was going through. The company you work for may or may not have an EAP. If they do, give them a try to see if it works for you.

5. **Praying and meditating:** Hospice work has a spiritual and sacred element. You may or may not have faith beliefs. If praying is a part of your daily life, then you already know its benefits. Praying can be a good outlet for expressing what is distressing you and then allowing you to release it. Meditation can also reduce stress and improve your emotional well-being. I know of team members who do this and find it beneficial to them.

6. **Personal memorial:** There is one thing that I do when one of my patients dies. I put a colored bead in a glass jar, take a small piece of paper, and write their name and what I remember most about them. I put that paper in the glass jar too. This has become a way to remember and release my patients.

I am sure there are other ways to process grief. These are only a few that have been beneficial to me. You might find other ways to process your grief.

How I Journal

Because I'm a natural writer, journaling is one of the best ways for me to process my work and the grief I am feeling. I write about the deaths of my patients and how they affected me, what I learned from caring for them, and what value I took away from the experience. In general, I write my experiences for the day, including the good, the bad, and the ugly. I write the things I've learned from my patients and things I want to do better—anything, really. Whatever comes to mind, I write it down.

I try to write every day, if possible. Some days, I just don't have the time or energy. But I find that writing something at the end of my day, even if it's a few sentences about my patients, helps me release the tensions I'm feeling. Often, I hold on to issues and problems, and all the details are constantly spinning around in my head. The act of writing them down helps me let go mentally, and it's actually a relief to do that.

Journaling will help you see how rich this hospice work is. Record your victories and what went right, your failures, and the things you could improve on. It gives you time to reflect instead of just going about your daily grind. I also recommend that you look back and read what you wrote a week or month before and see how you have grown. It really is an incredible process. You may discover some new things about yourself.

One More Thing

I recently talked with a former colleague, Mary Beth, an NP on our hospice team. She was always someone I could call and talk to about patients and coping with hospice work. As we remembered good times working together, she made a statement that I never thought about before during my hospice work. She said, "You have to be ok with your own mortality when working in hospice." I never thought I had to deal with that until I moved to southern Oregon and had quite a few patients who had cancer. Some of them were around my age and younger. Seeing those patients broke my heart. Especially the thirty-four-year-old mother who was dying of a rare brain cancer and she wasn't feeling well when I visited her. She had two rambunctious boys, full of energy and life, playing and running circles around her in the living room. It wasn't fair. I even felt like I had survivor's guilt. How was it that I got to live long enough to see my kids graduate from college, and she never will?

I really struggled with this issue of my own mortality. I had to journal about it for a long time to process and come to peace with the possibility of dying suddenly. What would I do if I was diagnosed with cancer myself? It was important for me to do this so that I could be prepared if that ever happened.

It also helped me reflect on my patients, be more compassionate with them, and be thankful for life.

In my quest to cope with my feelings when caring for young patients, the best advice I received was from one of our social workers, Lisa. She said that when you see a young patient, pretend that this is your last visit with them and make that moment count. Do all you can in that span of time to help that patient and care well for them. Somehow, that was very consoling. She was telling me I just had to give them my best, and I did.

THOUGHTS AND NOTES:

After reading this chapter, how will you do your grief work? How will you process it? It's necessary to have a plan. Try it out and see what works for you. Caring for your emotional health is a very important part of your work as a hospice nurse.

"And still, I rise." - Maya Angelou

A few months ago, I was talking with a former HMD, Dr. Shariff. I asked him what advice he would give to a new hospice nurse. He said, "You can learn something from every patient about life in general, not just about hospice. Things about relationships, mistakes, regrets." He also reminded me, "Every patient has a story to share."

SUNSET MEMORY

CHAPTER 14

FINDING CLOSURE

Another important thing to do in your hospice work is to find closure after the death of your patients. Doing this helps you tie loose ends in your experience with each patient and their families. Closure gives you a chance to remember, honor, and release the grief you have for your patients. How do you do this? There are several ways:

1. At (IDT) team meetings: During every team meeting, there is a bereavement time when the bereavement counselor will bring up the names of each patient who has died in the last two weeks since the last team meeting. As a nurse, you will be able to give a short overview of the care and death of the patient/family, and the other team members can share their experiences as well. This is not intended to be an in-depth discussion due to the time constraints of the IDT meeting, so you will need to keep your input brief and share the most important things. Usually, the social worker will notify the bereavement counselor if the family is having difficulty with the grieving process. This will inform the bereavement counselor to call the family earlier if they need grief support sooner.

2. A bereavement call: I usually make a bereavement call to the families two or three days after my patients die. The day of their loved one's death is usually too soon to call. There are exceptions, of course. Families usually go to the funeral home to make arrangements the next day. So, unless I think a family needs a bereavement call sooner rather than later, I usually wait. You will get a feel for when the time is right after you have done this several times. A bereavement call also gives you a chance to thank families for allowing you and your hospice team to care for

their loved one. This is usually when they would reciprocate and thank you for the good work you did in caring for their loved one. This can be a meaningful time and a good way to end your hospice relationship. It is the time when you may now step away from the family and allow them to grieve their loss. I always tell them that if they need help with anything, they should call our hospice office.

I found it's never too late to do a bereavement call. I remember once being so busy with work that I forgot to do a bereavement call to a family member. It was two or three weeks after the loved one had died. I felt bad that I had not contacted the family. I asked our bereavement counselor if it was too late to call, and she said no, that they would actually be grateful for the call, so I made it. And she was right, they were very happy I called. What a relief it was to me. It also gave me the closure I needed so I could go on.

3. Consider attending your patient's funeral if you are invited: Before the COVID pandemic, my team members and I used to attend as many funerals as we feasibly could, given our busy schedules. If the family members invited us to attend because we had developed a special connection over the time we cared for their loved ones, I usually went with the social worker and the LPN on our team.

   It was good for me because it allowed me to see patients in the progressive phases of life, from childhood to adulthood. Watching videos or looking at picture boards of them throughout their lifespan was heartwarming. I saw them young, vibrant, and full of life without illness or disease. It gave me a chance to celebrate the unique person they were and what they contributed to their community and the world. It was really an honor to attend my patients' funerals. The families would, in turn, appreciate us taking the time to attend and be present at their loved ones' memorial. The funerals I attended for my veteran patients at Arlington Cemetery were extra special. They were sacred and heartfelt tributes to our nation's heroes.

4. Annual bereavement programs or Ceremony of Remembrance services: This kind of service is held once a year. Some hospice companies, like the first one I worked for, have a memorial service planned by the hospice bereavement counselor. That counselor sent letters inviting family members to this service, usually held at a church or auditorium. The ones I attended included a formal program with candle lighting as the patients' names were announced. Family members would come

> up and light a candle in memory of their deceased loved one. A special song was played or sung, a poem was read, and a short talk was given at the end. After the service, there were refreshments and a time to meet family members, chat, and reminisce about their loved ones. Families enjoyed coming to these ceremonies and appreciated the time to remember their loved one in a special way.

Closure is important for hospice nurses. Doing this helps you reflect on your experiences, remembering all the good—and the bad—and seeing that everything turned out the best it possibly could in the end. Some of your patients and family dynamics will be a mess, and maybe you wish things had turned out differently. But there's no going back, so if a case is not ideal, you can still learn from it and go on. Then there are patients who die peacefully, and the family are thankful and at peace with everything. Cherish those times because it's not always going to be like that. Those are unforgettable memories that you will remember for a long time. Practice doing closure after your patients have died so that you can keep going forward and not get stuck in a grief cycle. If you need help to do this, ask your other team members. I know they would be more than happy to walk you through this.

THOUGHTS AND NOTES:

What ways do you think would help you process your work? Which ones mentioned above would you like to try?

"Nurses are there when the last breath is taken, and nurses are there when the first breath is taken. Although it is more enjoyable to celebrate the birth, it is just as important to comfort in death." - Christine Bell

I remember being invited to a funeral service at Arlington National Cemetery for one of my favorite patients, a high-ranking veteran. It was a well-attended service with a limo and a caisson (horse and carriage) escort. It was a sacred ceremony done with precision and timeliness, from the gun salute to the flag folding. The service was done with dignity, awe, and reverence for the deceased veteran and their family. It was such an honor to be there and witness that solemn occasion.

SUNSET MEMORY

CHAPTER 15

HOSPICE SURVEYS AND EVALUATIONS

CAHPS Hospice Survey

There is a Consumer Assessment of Healthcare Providers and Systems (CAHPS) hospice survey that is mailed to your patient's family or friend who knows the best about the hospice care provided by your hospice team. It is sent about two months after their loved one has died. It is a survey from the Centers for Medicare and Medicaid Services (CMS), which oversees hospice companies. It is an opportunity for family members to "grade" how you and your hospice team performed during their loved one's care. The responses result in a rating which is from one to five stars, with five stars being the highest. The ratings of all hospice companies in the U.S. are easily obtained on the internet. Just type Hospice Care Compare, and you will be directed to the Medicare.gov site to view all the hospice companies in the U.S.

This is a comprehensive survey that will cover different elements of hospice services. I would encourage you to look at this survey for yourself so you know what you and your team are being evaluated on. The survey can be found at this link: https://www.hospicecahpssurvey.org/. Use these questions to guide your work. The specific quality measures found below are what CMS is looking for to show hospice excellence. Patients and families will frequently research your hospice company to compare ratings of different hospice companies in your area before making a choice. As I mentioned, the higher your ratings, the more likely your company will be chosen. These star ratings are based on the scores from the CAHPS hospice surveys sent out.

According to Medicare, the survey information is gathered on six domains, including two global measures of care:

Here are the six domains or elements of the survey:

- Communication with family
- Getting timely help
- Treating patients with respect
- Emotional and spiritual support
- Help for pain and symptoms
- Training family to care for patient

There are two global measures of care:

- Rating of this hospice
- Willingness to recommend this hospice

These are sample questions on the survey:

Question #8: While your family member was in hospice care, how often did the hospice team explain things in a way that was easy to understand?

Question #14: How often did the hospice team listen carefully to you when you talked with them about problems with your family member's hospice care?

Question #16: Did your family member get as much help with pain as he or she needed?

If hospice team members perform well on these items, the CAHPS hospice star ratings can be elevated. Family members will usually choose the one with the highest rating. They want the best care possible for their loved ones. The reward for your hospice team when they work well together is a high rating, which may likely result in increased referrals of hospice patients to your company.

The one thing you can do to help your hospice team and the organization learn about what is going well, and what could be better, is to make sure that the right person is listed in the medical record to receive the survey. Sometimes, later in the hospice stay, it becomes clear to staff that the family member present at admission is not actually the person who is most likely to be with the patient during hospice visits. The person who is usually with you and the patient is the person who should receive the survey, even if they are "just" a friend or neighbor.

Your Hospice Company's Survey

If your hospice company desires to be accredited, an accrediting organization does an accreditation survey.

Community Health Accreditation Partner (CHAP) and The Joint Commission are common accrediting organizations, but others exist. If your organization chooses not to pursue accreditation but does accept payment from Medicare and Medicaid, the CMS, the state health authority, or a third-party contractor for one of these governmental bodies will conduct the survey.

The surveyors will look through random patient records to see if appropriate charting is done. They will go on visits with different team members and observe how they do their work. They typically will do this for about four or five days and then will give a final report at the end of their survey. They may also do remote record reviews but that will vary. At the end of the survey, they will recommend areas that need improvement.

This pertains to you because you should chart the appropriate things for your patients and make sure they are still appropriate for hospice services. Your charting should show that your patients are hospice-eligible. Remember that CMS believes the most important document is the care plan. I would advise that you learn how to chart care plans with detailed goals and outcomes.

If the surveyor accompanies you on one of your visits, it can be nerve-racking. But answer their questions to the best of your ability. They know you are new, so do the best work you can do on that visit. Also, be careful to follow your hospice company's hand washing and other hygiene policies. They may also inspect your trunk supplies and your nursing bag technique. Be sure to ask your nurse colleagues about these things. You will find that details of this hospice accreditation survey will frequently be discussed during IDT or RN meetings to prepare you for what is coming.

THOUGHTS AND NOTES:

During orientation, ask your clinical supervisor and nurse colleagues about these hospice surveys. Ask how you should prepare for them. What are the tips you should remember? Make a note of them here so you can refer to them later.

"Great things are not done by impulse, but by series of small things brought together." - Vincent van Gogh

When hospice CAHPS survey results are shared with your company they include comments from families. Versions of these will be sent from your clinical supervisor. Seeing family members mention you specifically to thank you for your outstanding care is very gratifying and will affirm that you made a difference in their lives.

SUNSET MEMORY

CHAPTER 16

THE GIFTS YOU GIVE

When I was new to hospice, I would describe myself as scared, tender, and sensitive. There was a LOT to learn, but I was up for the challenge. I didn't know what I was getting into. I saw and experienced things that made me very sad, and my tears flowed easily in the first year. It was hard work. But it got a little better as time went on. The more I learned about hospice, the more I began to treasure my experiences. My work became my identity. I drove myself to the limit, trying to do my best. In the beginning, I really had a hard time shutting work off, and I never really learned how to until years later. I came to a point where I realized I needed to care for myself more. I had to put work in its proper place in my life.

A former social work colleague, Faith, said hospice can be all-consuming. And she was right—if you let it. In this book, you might have noticed that I've focused a great deal on caring for yourself. Because you are constantly giving, you must take the time to rest, replenish, recover, renew, and restore yourself. Give yourself a buffer from work. You need to deliberately step away from it mentally and emotionally often, or it will indeed consume you. Nurture and nourish yourself as often as you can. Care for yourself as much as you care for your patients. Don't miss out on spending time with your family and friends. Recognize when it is time to take off your nurse hat and just be you. Yes, your work is important, and so are the gifts you give to them every day.

In your work as a hospice nurse, you will wonder what impact you are making. Sometimes, when you're so exhausted, you will wonder if you're doing anything at all. I want you to remember the following gifts you will give your patients daily.

Presence -This is the gift of just being with your patient; no words are needed. Your presence can provide comfort and calm for your patient.

Compassion - In this fast-paced world, you can offer deep and sincere compassion.

Patience - Sometimes, your patients will need to vent, or their family has a conflict. You can use your patience to help them work through their issues.

Listening - Learning to really listen to your patients and their families is an essential skill. Many family members have said that in their medical experience, they were not heard, so being a good listener is a valuable gift.

Time - When your patient has urgent needs or need some companionship, you will give them the gift of time.

Understanding - A daughter once thanked me for letting her talk about her frustrations with caregiving. She said her friends don't really understand what she's going through. You will provide that kind of understanding that others don't know how to give.

Who you are - The person you are is your gift to your patients. You will share the unique person you are through your past nursing and life experiences you've had,

Gentleness - There are tender moments when your patients will need your gentle touch and words. They will appreciate you for your gentleness in their anxious and fearful moments.

Healing - Healing can take different forms for patients and their families. Healing in relationships, spiritual healing, and emotional healing are some of the ways you can provide healing.

Respect - Honoring and respecting your patients' end-of-life wishes is a huge gift to them and their families.

Comfort - You have the opportunity to provide physical and emotional comfort at every visit. This is especially needed when a patient is declining and requires symptom management or when your patient is at EOL.

Acceptance - One patient who had breast cancer showed me her disfigured chest area after she had surgery. I allowed her to express her feelings of horror and told her that I accepted her just as she was and gave her a sense of peace. You will do that, too.

No matter what kind of days you have, I want you to know how valuable you are to everyone you work with, including your team. Like I've said before, the things you do for your patients and their families will be remembered forever. As you remember your patients after they have died, remember the gifts you have given them and the gifts they have given you. Cherish the hospice team you are part of, and know that thousands of hospice nurses all over the U.S. are providing this compassionate end-of-life care.

On my hard days, I've come very close to quitting. I can't tell you how many times I said this to myself and my teammates; I don't know how much longer I can do this. And ironically, on those days, a patient and family member expressed their thanks and gratitude for being there for them. I remember a patient's wife who told me on a particularly difficult day, "I'm proud of you," as I cared for her husband. She had no idea how her simple compliment had pulled me out of the pit of discouragement. This will happen to you too. Just when you least expect it, you will get words of affirmation from your patient, a family member, or your fellow team member. And that's what will keep you going, knowing that your efforts have not been in vain.

Whenever I get any positive comments during my visits, I write them down. I encourage you to do the same. Put them in your journal. That way, you'll be able to look back and see the evidence that you did something meaningful—something good in the world. It will be a gift to yourself. Enjoy this position as a hospice nurse and a sunset angel. Like I said in the beginning, I believed in you then, and now believe in you even more so as you have finished reading this book. You now know what I have learned. I hope you feel more prepared and equipped to do this hospice work. What you experience in this position will significantly impact your nursing career and your personal life.

So, I end by saying to you, as my hospice mentor, Sheila, used to say to me, "Now go out there and make a difference!"

As long as I am sharing words of wisdom, I want to share one of my all-time favorite poems by John Greenleaf Whittier. I kept it on my wall when I was in nursing school, and reading it kept me going. You may have heard it before, but I wanted you to have it handy to remind you not to quit.

DON'T QUIT

When things go wrong as they sometimes will,
When the road you're trudging seems all up hill,
When the funds are low and the debts are high
And you want to smile, but you have to sigh,
When care is pressing you down a bit,
Rest if you must, but don't you quit.

Life is strange with its twists and turns
As every one of us sometimes learns
And many a failure comes about
When he might have won had he stuck it out;
Don't give up though the pace seems slow —
You may succeed with another blow.

Success is failure turned inside out—
The silver tint of the clouds of doubt,
And you never can tell just how close you are,
It may be near when it seems so far;
So stick to the fight when you're hardest hit—
It's when things seem worst that you must not quit.

For all the sad words of tongue or pen
The saddest are these: "It might have been!"

- John Greenleaf Whittier
(1807-1892)

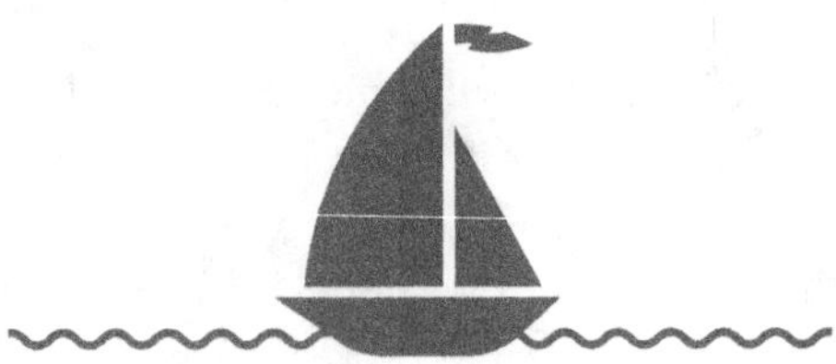

CHAPTER 17

TOOLS AND RESOURCES

This is a list of professional and self-care resources I thought you might find useful and practical for work and personal growth. You might come across other resources that you can add to this list. Ask your hospice team what resources they would recommend. This will enrich your life and your work.

Books:
Hospice Quickflips© for NGS is an essential reference booklet for hospice RN case managers. *Fast Facts for the Hospice Nurse* - This book is one that every clinical supervisor has given me in the different hospice companies I've worked for. You will most likely get this book, too. *The Helper's Journey* by Dale G. Larson, who is a former bereavement counselor. I used to read this book for our centering moment to teach us to be an effective helper to those facing grief and loss.

Certified Hospice and Palliative Nurse (CHPN) - After three or four years of hospice work, consider getting your hospice certification. You may also opt to get it sooner; it just depends on your readiness. When you sense that you are more confident and competent with your skills as a hospice nurse, start studying for this certification. Get a CHPN prep book and find apps with sample questions to help you prepare for this exam. It takes a few months of studying to fully understand how to take this test and what to expect. In the end, you will feel a sense of accomplishment. This will help your career as a hospice nurse, and most companies will increase pay as well.

The book that I used was the *Certified Hospice and Palliative Nurse (CHPN) Exam Review* by Patricia Moyle Wright. There are many books and apps out there to help you prepare for this exam. The main app that I used the most was the CHPN Practice Test app, which is free in your app store. Every day, I would get test questions, and it would give me a percentage grade and show me my weaknesses and what I needed to study more.

These are the resources that I have used to help me on my hospice journey:

- Facebook - Hospice Nursing Support Group. You can ask just about any question regarding your hospice work. This is a safe place, to be honest about your frustrations or just to ask for help solving a problem. You can glean knowledge from the more experienced nurses. You'll find encouragement and practical information in this group.
- The Art of Listening in a Healing Way by James E. Miller.- This is a short and easy-read book written by a grief counselor. You will learn the skill of true listening.
- Podcasts by hospice nurse James Dibben, RN. He also has a website called Confessions of a Hospice Nurse.
- Hospice Nurse Hero. Online support by Rochelle Hobson, RN, MSN, CHPN.

Books about self-care:

- *Simple Self-Care for Therapists* by Ashley Davis Bush. I was introduced to this book through a former bereavement counselor, Dianne. She had read sections from this book. It has short, easy, and often fun exercises you can do to help restore and renew your physical and emotional energies.
- *The Self-Care Prescription* by Robyn L Gobin, PhD. This is a valuable book on self care in every aspect of your life. It is colorful and fun to read.
- *Restore: 20 Self-Care Rituals to Reclaim Your Energy* by The Essentialists.
- *A Book That Loves You: An Adventure in Self-Compassion* by Irene Smit and Astrid Van Der Hulst.
- *Positive Affirmations for Women* by Grace Law. Affirmations are just the thing to give you a lift at the start of your day and throughout the day.
- *The Complete Guide to Self Care: Best Practices for a Healthier and Happier You* by Kiki Ely.
- *Compassion Fatigue* by Beverly Kyer.
- *Sabbath: Finding rest, renewal, and delight in our busy lives* by Wayne Muller. A former bereavement counselor, Dianne Henry-Legget, read an excerpt from this book during the IDT meeting, and afterward, I knew I had to get my own copy.

MY DAILY VISIT WORKSHEET

In my first year of hospice work, I created a worksheet because I was tired of forgetting important things during my visits. This form is a work in progress. Over time, I have changed a few things here and there when I think it would be more beneficial for me during my visits. So, use this as an example, and feel free to tweak it to your liking and make it your own.

Date__________ Mileage __________

Start Time________ End Time ________

Name _________________ Age ______

Dx ______________________________

VS: T____ P____ (R/Irreg) R____ BP____

Resp: CTA____ Dim____ Crackles____

Wheezing ____ Cough____ SOB_____

Abd: Soft___ NT___+/-BS___ LBM_____

MAC (mid arm cir) R_______ L________

Pain: Located _____________________

PAIN AD ____ Self Report ____ Rate____

Mental status/physical appearance _______

____

Main problem: ____________________

____

PO intake: ___________ Appetite_______

Feeds self: ____ Time takes to feed pt:____

Cardiac: CP__Murmur__Tachy__Brady__

Skin: ___________________________

Mobility: ________________________

Wound(s)

Location_________ Location_________

Drainage_________ Drainage_________

Measurement______ Measurement______

Type____________ Type____________

NOTES:

Call family for update____ Faxed note to facility___ New orders:

ABOUT THE AUTHOR

ELLEN G. MORGAN, RN, BSN, CHPN

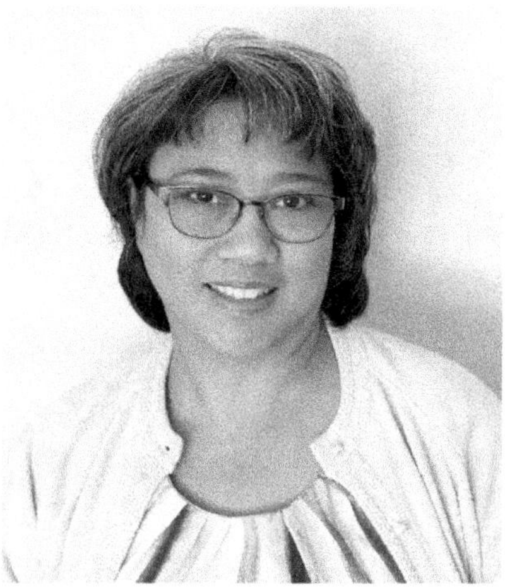

Thank you so much for reading this book. I wrote it for you—to help you as a new hospice nurse survive and succeed in your career. I want it to be a source of encouragement and hope—a companion to help guide you through the beginning days of your new journey. I have committed myself to support and motivate hospice nurses to keep going.

I want you to know that becoming a hospice nurse is a noble career choice and that you don't have to navigate the journey on your own.

I've been an RN for thirty years and a hospice nurse for eleven of those years. People have asked me many times how I do this kind of work. I usually acknowledge the difficulty of this work. But then I say that hospice is a celebration of life and a way to honor patients' life contributions to society. There is joy in hospice, too.

I would describe myself as creative, quiet, fun, gentle, and kind. I am a lover of a good challenge, a fierce advocate for my patients, am musical and crafty, and enjoy cooking. I am also a chocoholic. I am a woman of detail but also have an easygoing personality. My husband, Dwight, and I reside in southern Oregon and have three beautiful adult daughters and two grandchildren. I love crafts of any kind, am an avid Audible reader/listener, a novice quilter, and a nature photographer.

For questions, please email me at writingnurse270@gmail.com or find me on my website at ellengmorgan.com.

All the best,
Ellen

GRATITUDE

Where do I start to thank those who have encouraged me to write this book? I could not have done it without God's guidance, who led me to the right people to work with. He also gave me the wisdom and courage to step forward into this realm of writing, and I want to thank Him with all my heart.

Thank you to my very supportive husband, Dwight, who never stopped encouraging me and telling me to keep going in this book endeavor. I am also grateful to my family and friends who supported me along this writing journey. I love you all!

Kent Sanders, founder of Profitable Writers. Thank you for giving me such good advice when I needed it. You showed me that it is possible to make a living as a writer, which has been a longtime dream of mine.

I also want to thank my editor, Karen Hunsanger, who has been my cheerleader every step of the way. I have leaned on your guidance, which has helped me grow as a writer.

Thank you to my proofreader, Rick Fordyce, for your keen eye for detail.

I am so appreciative of Kaycee Parker's work as my graphic designer. She came through for me in her creative work on the book cover and interior design. Your stunning work brought me to tears when I first saw it.

I would like to thank my beta readers for generously giving their time. Mayple Lynx, Rochelle Webster, NP, Claire Hart, Rebecca Conrad, and Wanita Toews, you are very much appreciated.

Last but not least, these are hospice colleagues, former and current, who I would like to thank for their special contributions to this book:

Dr. Imran Shariff, Mary Beth Reckmeyer-Armstrong, Denise Smith, Faith Brown-Edwards, Joyce Montgomery, Dawn Watt, Rochelle Webster, Sheila Lax, Arion Lillard-Green, Patricia Lyle, Kathleen Buday, Dianne Henry Leggett, Mike Ridge, Mino Isopescu, Audrey O'Donoghue, Lisa Allred and Richard Evans.

www.ingramcontent.com/pod-product-compliance
Lightning Source LLC
LaVergne TN
LVHW022228200926
848481LV00006B/2169
* 9 7 9 8 9 9 1 8 8 0 4 0 4 *